___ Do Me!

Stefan Müller, born in Munich in 1961, has worked exclusively as a writer for television (*Marienhof, Soko,* as well as numerous courtroom shows and entertainment programs) and as a journalist writing about the gay scene. His writings for Bruno Gmünder include a portrait of the city of Munich in *Männer* magazine and the city guide *München von hinten.* At present, he works in management (in the field of market research) and only occasionally writes for less hectic and more pleasurable projects than anything the infotainment sector has to offer. His short stories are currently available in *Die Nacht und ich* (Bruno Gmünder) and *Hiebe & Triebe 5* (Querverlag).

Stefan Müller

DO ME!

The Complete Guide to Adventurous Gay Sex

BRUNO GMÜNDER

Disclaimer:
The writer and publisher encourage you to be aware that you are taking some risk when you engage in sexual activities. Neither the author, the publisher, nor anyone else associated with the creation or sale of this book is responsible for any injuries sustained.

DO ME!

1st edition
Copyright © 2014 Bruno Gmünder Verlag GmbH, Germany
Original title: Besorg's mir! Der schwule Sex-Ratgeber
für Fortgeschrittene
Text: © Stefan Müller
Translation: Nicola Heine
Cover art: Dolph Caesar
Cover photo: © Dylan Rosser; www.dylanrosser.com
Layout: Enrico Dreher
Photo credits: page 168

Bruno Gmünder Verlag GmbH
Kleiststraße 23-26, 10787 Berlin
info@brunogmuender.com

Printed in Germany

ISBN 978-3-86787-692-6

More about our books and authors:
www.brunogmuender.com

Imagination does not mean inventing things,
it means caring about them.
—Thomas Mann

CONTENTS

Rituals and Signals 37

Master of the Senses 60

A Recipe for Good Sex (Ingredients) 97

Preface

*The secret of happiness is freedom
and the secret of freedom is courage.*
—Pericles of Athens

Men are amazing. Sex is amazing. Sex with men, from brief quickies
to entire sex marathons, is incredibly amazing. It is a well-known
fact that time does not determine quality, for sometimes the memory
of a brief encounter will linger on forever in our minds and loins.
From time to time, I find it difficult to analyze the quality, as I quite
frequently have no idea why one encounter feels more intense to me
than another. However, sometimes I can pinpoint exactly why the
sex was so good. The following guide is about this kind of good sex.
I wish I had good sex more of the time, but at least I have an idea
of how it ought to be and what it needs to include: the right combination of respect and selfishness, movement and standstill, dominance and submission, pleasure and pain, concentration and ecstasy.
Sticking it in is still one of high points, but you should also try out
other sensations, too—after all, in adult gay sex, anything enjoyable
goes. A wider repertoire can be applied with equal success during a
quickie with an unknown but incredibly hot guy if the right signals
are sent and received clearly—and that's a learning process!—but it
will work out even better with a man you already know, for trust is
an important key to carrying out the more complicated and intense
sex games, just as important as understanding and accepting rules.
Just like real life.

This guide is meant not so much for specialists of particular fields
such as bondage or S&M, but rather for anyone interested in playing with variations, for gay men who are sexually active with their
partners or in the scene and would like to spice up their sex lives.
It is even less suitable for prudes. May they play with their dicks in
peace and quiet until they finally find eternal rest. This is for men,

young and old, who are really into men—from head to toe! Your willingness to savor the length and breadth of passion between men should be driven by more than curiosity. You should be really into it!

I'm assuming you've picked this book up out of curiosity as to whether you might be tempted by the occasional scenario suggested here. If your sex life has given no cause for complaints up to now, so much the better. Subjecting yourself to pressure (for example, the idea that you need to be better than the competition) should not be the reason for reading this book.

The suggestions you will find in this book are *examples* and have not always been followed to completion, as sex never follows a pre-written script. I've included a couple of short sex stories here and there to demonstrate the practical application of the respective chapters and hopefully to whet your appetite. Over the course of reading, you will get to know the two couples featured here. They will certainly offer lots of suggestions on how to continue the stories and to create your own variations using your imagination. As you've all had—or would like to have—your own exciting and unusual fantasies, I would be delighted if you felt like sharing any anecdotes or suggestions for improving any of the chapters with me, care of the publisher, Bruno Gmünder Verlag. After all, there's room for improvement in my sex life, too!

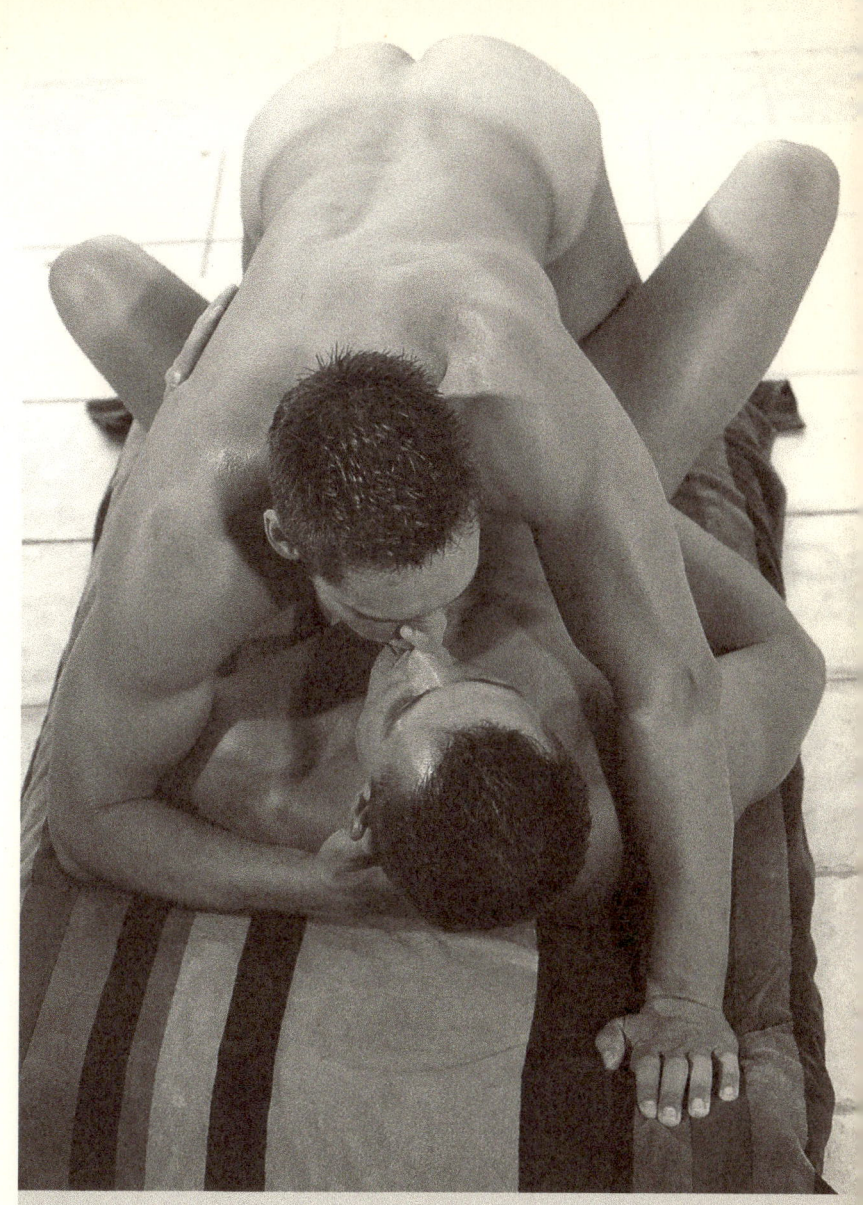

Savoring the length and breadth of passion

13

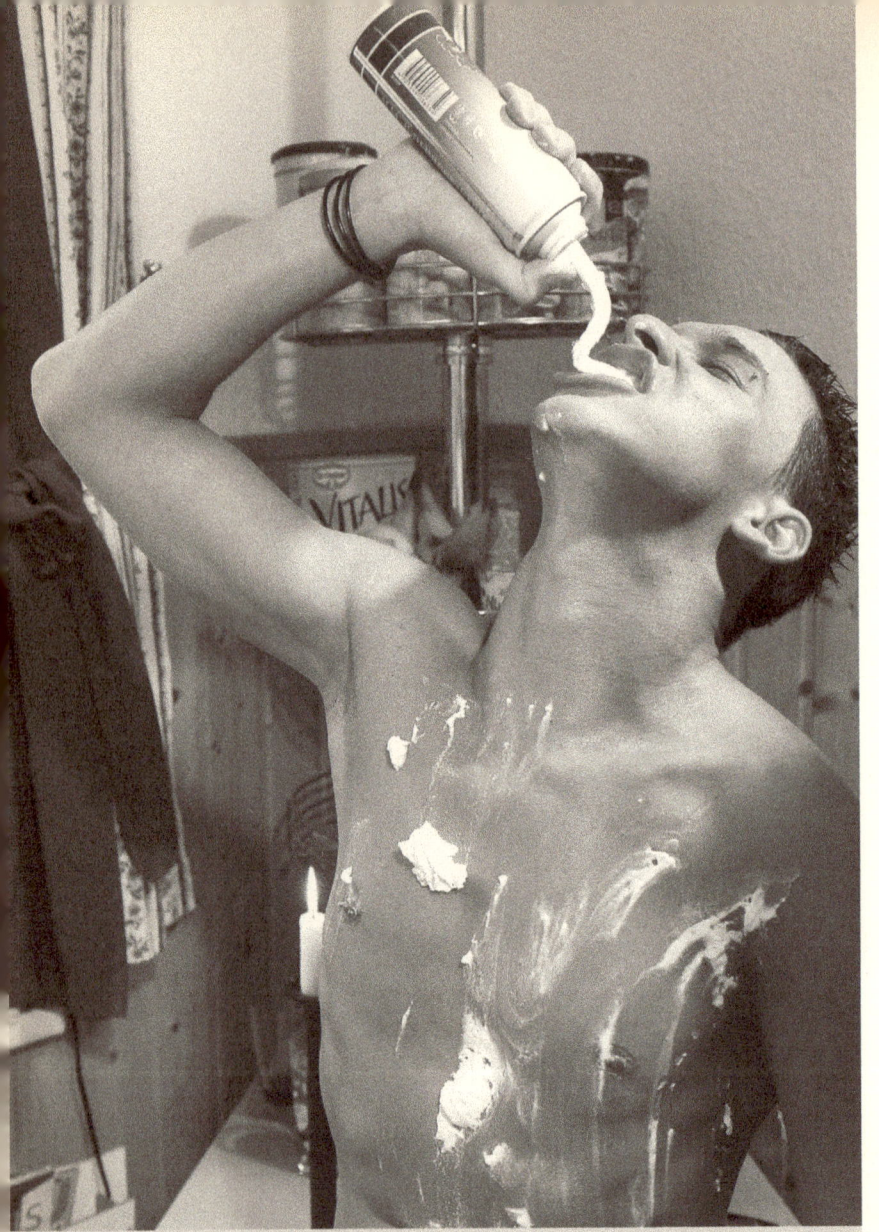

Sex with a man tastes so much better!

Really Good Sex

▼ Sex and Sex

Our real and virtual worlds can cater to nearly every fantasy—all you need is the appropriate place or media. Putting too much pressure on yourself can drive you insane. But in my experience, one single intense encounter can make you so much happier than a hundred insignificant fucks, so why all the pressure? Once you've stepped out of the numbers race, you can kick back and wait for your next opportunity. Your own comfort is more important than any film, book, or story that tries to make you believe in the perfect and everlasting orgasm. I've nothing against blowing off steam by indulging in the occasional no-strings-attached sex, though. If you have better sex with yourself than with another man, those aren't grounds for resignation, but after reading this book you will hopefully be inspired to find out once more how sex with a man tastes!

Good sex works best if the liberties you take are in harmony with your conscience. Great sex and a guilty conscience are *not* compatible. Before you pass judgment on your own fantasies or those of your partner, you might want to ask yourself why. Upbringing, moral values, health risks, fears—all of these may affect whether or not you can enjoy the sex you want without regret. Guilt is a terrible erotic stimulus. Once you are aware of and have accepted your own sexuality, only then can you transfer your own pleasure to your partner. Only then will you really be able to enjoy sex. The more cheerfully you act out your sexuality, the easier it will be to sweep your partner along.

▼ Planned or Spontaneous?

Really good sex isn't mass-produced, it's an exquisite experience. It has nothing to do with the everyday fare you eat to satisfy your hunger—that's why it should be experienced in reasonable doses. But you should treat yourself to a proper helping once in a while!

Greed is completely inappropriate here. Enjoyment takes priority. Practice the art of limitation: Just lie back and feel every kiss, every fuck, every blow of the whip. Each one of these can be an incredible experience. You are under no obligation to work your way through the entire range—that is not an indication of quality. Feeling hungry is enough to turn sex into *really good* sex, although a whetted appetite will usually do it, too.

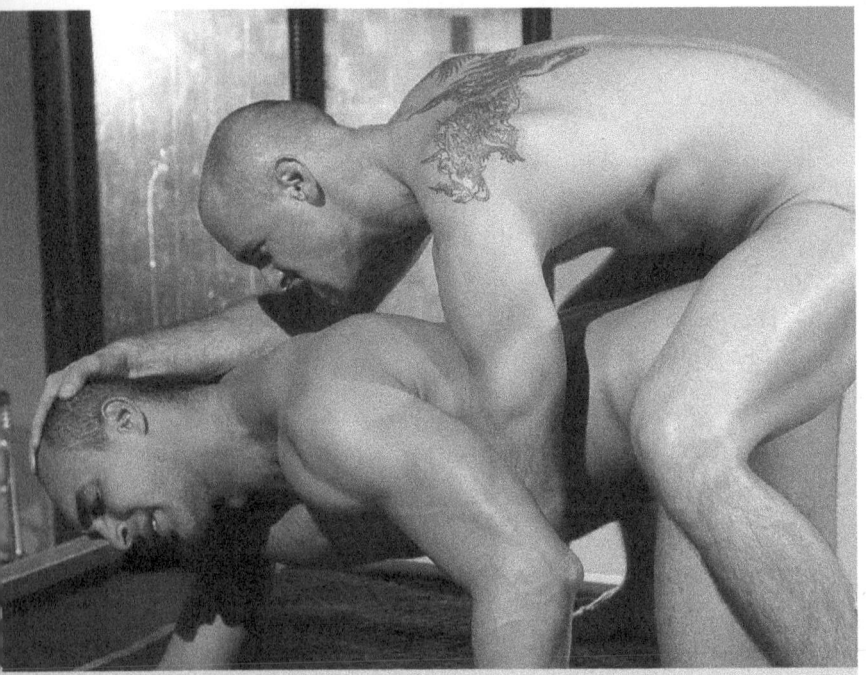

Sitting back is not always easy.

While we're on the subject: if your stomach is full, your body will be occupied with matters other than sexual challenges. Feeling full can place a burden on passion. Add to that the fact that some of your orifices might be needed something other than evacuation. If you're full to the brim at both ends, accidents can happen that will kill the mood. If sex is in the cards, it's best to tighten your belt. So, don't stuff yourself—eat sensibly, eat something that will increase your sense of well-being instead. This can become part of prepping your body for some action. Fruit, a steak, carbs, seafood, a milkshake? Every body has its own particular combination that makes it feel good. If you want to approach your inner animal in spirit, eating raw meat—for example, carpaccio or raw fish—counts as a legitimate way of doing it. Bon appétit!

Consciously savoring sex with another man is even more enjoyable if you plan it first. It's like preparing a really good dinner: planning, shopping, cooking. And then eating it! Of course, the question is: Are you both ordering from the same menu?

▼ Male Fantasies

Any sexual fantasy that comes to mind should first be approached conceptually. The easiest way of finding out whether or not something you haven't done yet turns you on is by playing it out by yourself—that is to say, while jerking off. So whenever you're in the middle of a solo session, try letting a fantasy you've been entertaining for a long (or short) while approach. You'll find out soon enough whether it heightens or impedes your arousal. Even if a fantasy turns you on now, that does not necessarily mean you need to put it into practice. But it's conceivable. As long as it's legal, you can confidently go about bringing it to fruition.

No matter how innocent or dirty your fantasy may be, there is no need to be alarmed by it. I can guarantee that you are not the only person to have entertained something of the kind during a randy moment. Men like to be heroes but, as you may have noticed during the course of your life, they also like to be pigs. They have incredibly dirty thoughts. Be assured: The man you're currently getting busy with—or are about to—has depths that are just as abysmal as your own! That comes with the territory of being a man. And you're no exception. There's no need to feign shame! That's the great thing about being gay. Welcome to a man's world! You can get quite an accurate impression of this world by watching a straight porno. Those guys fuck with a helping of selfishness that's miles away from shamefaced insecurity. They don't seem to be at all worried about whether their partners like them or what their partners are feeling at the moment, and they aren't even interested in finding out. So, they just kick off or lie back and let themselves be serviced. Shouldn't sex between men be even less complicated?

As a gay man, you should be familiar with your partner's bodily setup—after all, he's a man, too. Both men ought to be able celebrate what they have in common—that's way more fun than looking for the differences. So, why not act fearlessly, rather than inhibit yourself with the faulty assumption that you are having sex with an unknown entity?

Sex can only be really hot once you accept that things can be beautifully uncomplicated when you're both playing at the same level. Then you can start getting down and dirty. We may wish to be gods, but our animalistic side is a much greater source of happiness, passion, and pleasure. People—not just men—are simply animals. We tiptoe around our sexual needs, afraid to plumb those depths that might, in another context, be unappetizing. Slipping into that noble pelt, diving into the depths of carnal lust will ground you and give you the strength to soar.

Drop your inhibitions and live your dreams! You can do it quickly, at a moment's notice, or gradually, slowly, and carefully, as if stalking your prey. The important thing is the desire to do it!

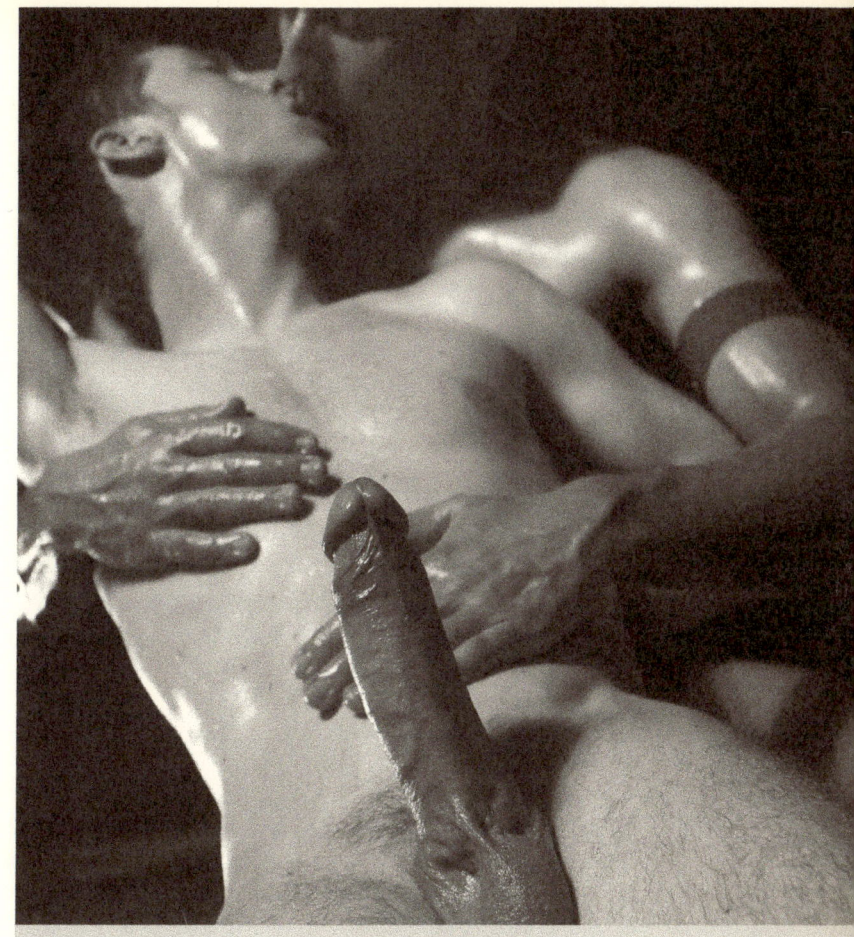

Drop your inhibitions and reach for this.

▼ Safe, Sane, Consensual

There are a couple of basic conditions for a happy and successful sexual adventure. One important rule is that sex should be "SSC": *safe, sane, and consensual*. These three words, the holy trinity of S&M, also apply to any form of sexual congress.

Sex doesn't just cover what's happening with your dick or your ass at a given moment, but principally what's happening in your gut and in your head. Both your physical and mental well-being are important. Without them, you won't really enjoy shooting your load.

Safe refers not only to the rules of safe sex, reformulated here in our chapter on *Safer Sex*, but also to overall physical, mental, and emotional safety. Your partner needs to know that he can have sex with you without damage to body or soul.

Sane may sound boring, and is possibly an elastic term, but basically everyone knows what the word means.

Consensual means that both partners have to give their consent. The opposite of that is rape. If you can't manage to entice your partner towards a particular sexual fantasy so that he actually wants to do it, you'll have to come up with something else.

Either this book will help you find arguments to interest him in your fantasy, or it will give you some alternatives that both of you will enjoy just as much. Or possibly even more.

▼ Ground Rule: Respect

Now for some moralizing, for the first and only time in this book. An important requirement for using the tips and tricks listed here is respect for your partner and for yourself. If your sex life is such that you can't look at yourself in the mirror after at least one out of three tricks, then something is very wrong. Even if you're crawling out of the darkroom or your bedroom on all fours, your moral self has to remain upright, otherwise it will break you down. What turns you on or not doesn't depend on the external action, but rather on the internal stance you take, no matter whether you're into humiliation, degradation, anonymity, or pain. As long as you can pleasurably incorporate it into your sex life, it's all good. That doesn't mean you have to go along with everything. If you feel like a stranger to

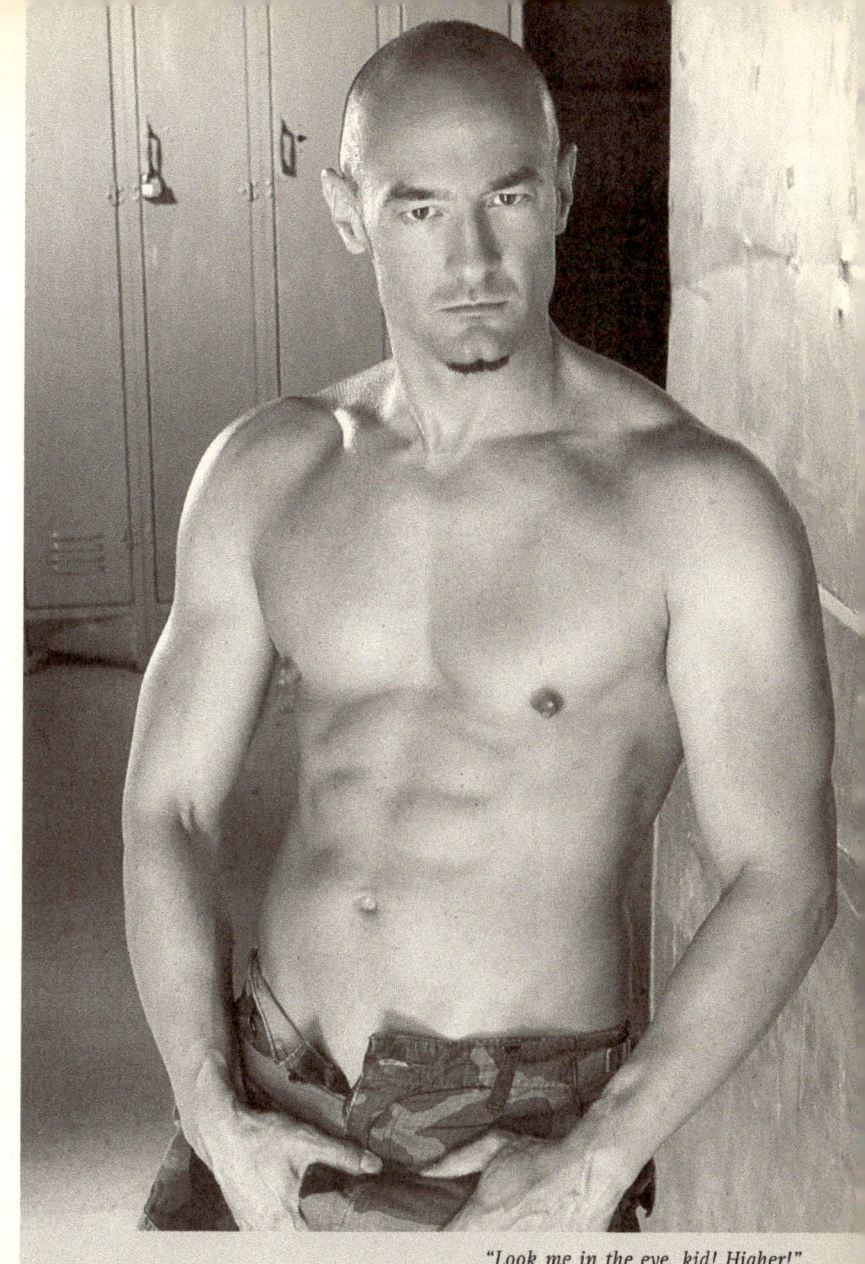

"Look me in the eye, kid! Higher!"

21

yourself afterwards, if you're sad or distraught over a longer period of time, then it's high time to rethink your sex life. Above all: Don't let anyone violate your personal integrity and don't violate any else's! However rough and dirty you want to play, there has to be enough time and the opportunity to regain your balance, during or after sex, on your own or as a couple. You don't have to understand or accept everything that happens, but you must never lose sight of your mutual respect, otherwise you'll have to say good-bye to your dreams of good sex.

Even if the sex isn't going too well or there's an accident, you can still treat each other with respect. There is no need to be rude if your partner wants to do something you don't understand or want. If you have learned to grasp and accept yourself as a unique individual, you can also concede to the other guy's uniqueness and difference.

If you get the feeling that your sex partner is an asshole who doesn't respect you or if you don't respect him, then hands off! There are plenty of other men you can have sex with!

The Right Man

Whenever a couple on a TV show has problems in bed, a friend
or professional counselor always advises the affected party to "Try
wearing the—alternately—red, black, or short dress! That will really
turn him on!" If it were only that easy! I don't think it's enough to
just hit the right button in order to suddenly have incredibly hot
sex with the same partner you've just been letting off steam with up
till now. Men are—thank God!—complex beings. Let's say you have
piss-related fantasies. So far, you've never brought this up with your
boyfriend, never even hinted at them. Besides the fact that our fantasies are linked to various types of men—the skinhead, the rascal, the
cutie, the slut—your guy will always be the man you first consciously
or unconsciously saw him as. You don't want to be pissed on by
him, even in a red garter belt. (Especially not in a red garter belt!)
Then you're going to have to either forget about this fantasy (after
all, there are more important things than piss), or else try it out with
someone else. You might not have any trouble carrying out your
golden shower fantasies with another man. You can't have every
kind of sex with every man. But after all, this is about having good
sex, not about acting out a specific fantasy. If the two coincide, so
much the better! So, it's not about finding the right man, but rather
about doing the right thing with the man you're with at the moment,
provided that you want to do it with him, of course. That should be
enough. If you decide right now that you want to have really good
sex, you can do that.

Men are so full of surprises and so exciting that fixating on a single
fraction of them is a pointless waste, a self-imposed loss. The guy
you're currently involved with has heaps of secrets for you to discover, even if you've known him for years. If you're having sex, there
has to be some intimacy between you—not just physical closeness,

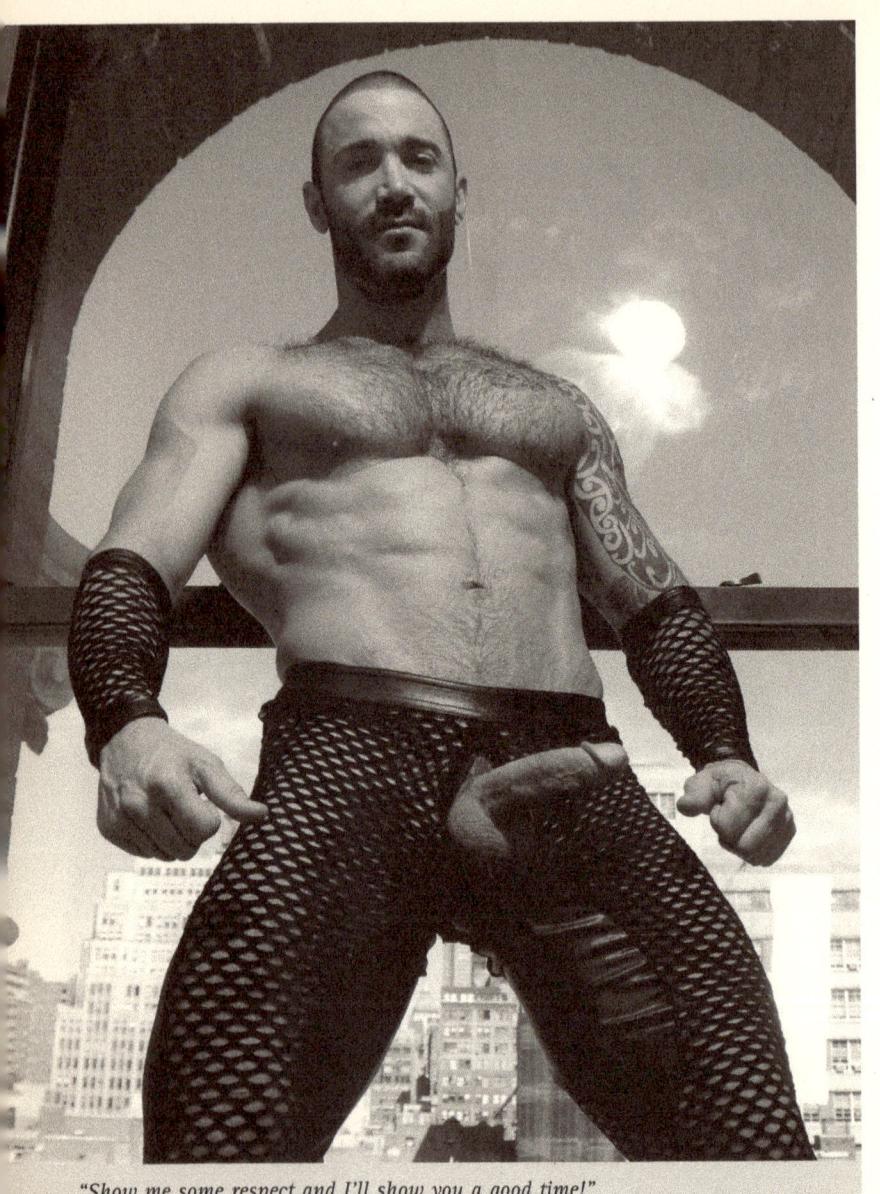

"Show me some respect and I'll show you a good time!"

but also the willingness to open up to each other mentally. Intimacy creates a framework for getting to know your partner's sexuality anew, or once again, but from a different perspective. Blessed are those who are able to shift their focus and come up with new ideas to get closer to their partners again and again. You don't necessary have to get physical right away. After all, sex takes place mainly inside your head. His thoughts and your thoughts are important—every kiss, every touch can summon up mental images to stimulate both of you sexually. You can exchange them, whisper them, or show them to each other. The path towards good sex has to be taken together—it involves a combination of leading, stopping, waiting, and following. Sending signals is important—these are your signposts. If your partner doesn't understand your signals, you can't have good sex with him. Good communication is key here. More on that in the upcoming chapters.

▼ Second Scenario: The Stranger

Sex with strangers can be an incredibly joyless affair. But an encounter with a perfect stranger can also all of a sudden make you step outside boundaries you have never crossed before, whether with your previous partner or with anyone else. Every gay man has access to plenty of guys and opportunities for experimentation—these can all be found in the customary places and media. As long as you stick to the ground rules (see above: respect!), you can generally rule out doing any lasting harm by experimenting. If you are seriously interested in certain sexual practices and the opportunity arises or catches you off-guard—go for it! Don't worry, your reputation won't be damaged by one small foray into an exotic sexual practice. Even if your little adventure does make the gossip rounds, in the world of gay erotica it will be just an anecdote at best—so what? It's better than waiting forever and then being annoyed with yourself for not having tried it out before. You don't know this guy, you don't know the slightest thing about him, he is merely the instrument of your lust. So help yourself! If you want something specific from him, there are plenty of ways to show him.

Are You Up for Some Really Good Sex?

If you want to experience great sex, you have to sweep your partner off his feet or let yourself be swept away. That's the great thing about spontaneous sex, you don't get the chance to deliberate. You go out, take things as they come, and *boom!* You're swept off your feet! But what if you're planning on having sex?

If you're not comfortable with yourself, cheerful sex is going to be hard to accomplish. It's a bit much to expect your partner to change your mood for you. But you really want sex now? If you've made up your mind to step up to the sexual stage even though you're not feeling too great, you should first try and improve your mood.

If it's just a passing state of mind you're aware of but don't want it to stop you from hooking up with someone, you'll probably know one or two ways of getting yourself in the right mood. In any case, you should try to alleviate your stress in order for it to clear a space for anticipation, so that it can grow and let desire lead your spirits back on the right track.

If your mind is already on track, you need to make your body follow. It isn't easy to be happy with your own body, at least for most of us, especially if you're letting some dumb mirror set the standard. But since you already know how to pay attention to another man's sexiness, there's no need for harsh criticism. It doesn't matter how old you are, how fat or how thin, it matters how you present yourself. Your personality is what counts. What do you want? Show what you want, as best you can! If you don't express yourself, you won't get what you want.

This applies just as much to sex as to real life: The more you're aware of the relationship between the makeup, the costume, and your lines, the better you will be able to play your role, and the more successful the play will be.

That doesn't mean you have to renounce your personality and pretend to be someone you're not—on the contrary: be yourself! Apart

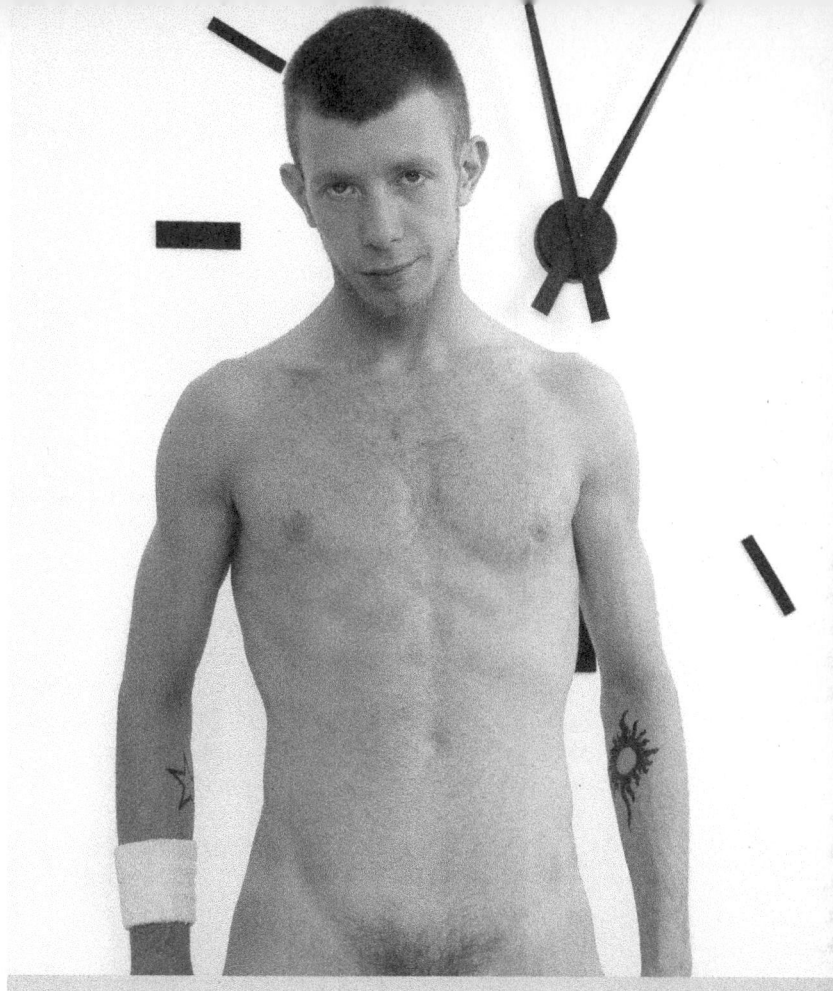

"What time is it? Sex o'clock!"

from the teeming chaos created by the innumerable characters of the millions of people around you and farther afield, every single one of them also has widely different temperaments and characteristics. All kind of men see all kinds of other men as hot. The important thing is to show who and what you are and what you want. You may find a dress code on how to send out the right sexual signals helpful (see *Sending Signals—Sex and Clothing*).

External Circumstances

Apart from your momentary emotional state and physical actions, there are plenty of external circumstances that make up the requirements for an intense and lasting experience. You won't have the opportunity to use that many tricks during a quickie in a hotel elevator, but the electric atmosphere still may create a memory that's hotter than most others. The location, setting, light, sounds, or music can stimulate and inspire your imagination, as can certain clothes and accessories. You can certainly influence these factors by making conscious choices.

The problem, however, is that these choices, in order to remain impressive in the sense of being imprinted in our conscious mind, can never or rarely be repeated, otherwise the impression will wear thin and will no longer make much of an impact. It will become at best a ritual that increases your anticipation for something familiar, for example always putting the same dildo in the same place. It should *not* become a routine. You can change the precise moment in time when you decide to use it. You can change the length of time you use it for. What the hell—you can always buy another one in a different color! Surprises are a good way of creating a lasting impression. As I have just described, there are a few simple tricks you can use to create a change that will throw a new light on something familiar and turn it into something fresh and new. You'll find a couple of examples in the next chapter.

Once you've decided to try out a concrete fantasy on a particular night, you can give it a try in public at a fetish party or a club. Handcuffs attached to your belt in the right place, wearing the appropriate hanky in your pants pocket or around your neck, a slave collar, rubber, leather—there are many items of clothing and accessories that will make the wearer's desires apparent. Warning: The signals you send will be taken seriously here! See the chapter on *Rituals and Signals* for an explanation of what they mean.

They stand for certain intentions in the same way, whether you wear them in private or leave them lying out at home. If you open the door to your partner naked, that can of course be a signal, too. The right choice of clothing is definitely a part of getting yourself in the mood for a sexual adventure, so it can't hurt to pay attention to this point before you get going. It stands to reason that you won't find the right men unless you are yourself and show everyone who you are, doesn't it?

▼ The Right Setting for Good Sex

Gritty cruising area, stylish loft, country style apartment—great sex can be had anywhere. The setting depends on your personal taste. It doesn't matter where the action takes place, only how. The right atmosphere can, however, play a part in guiding your sexual fantasies in a certain direction.

Gay men are just as inventive as straight couples when it comes to choosing a location to have sex in: on board a plane, on a construction site or a beach, in a cheap hotel as well as the standard settings, such as the sauna, the darkroom, the men's room, professional playrooms or porn movie theaters. The places we've just listed owe a good part of their sex appeal to their neutrality. They have nothing to do with the participants' personalities and so they are neutral territory. None of the dirt, smells, appurtenances, or positive or negative attributes will be linked to either you or your partner.

But what about your own private apartment? Good sex is not tied to good taste, so that ought to be a relief for some of us. Your home is very likely suitable for sex, but depending on your own sexual preferences, you should always take a close look at the setting, not just when you're expecting a blind date. It will also be easier to seduce your long-term partner into having really good sex if you first take a quick look around you.

For instance, is there anything lying around that could be construed as the opposite of sexy? Disgusting (used Q-tips), depressing (your last bank statement), or too private (that party photo that shows you lying asleep on the couch, drunk, drooling, and having pissed your pants)? When having spontaneous sex, changing positions and coming face to face with a prescription for the abscess cream your current sex partner appears to be using at the time may at best be interpreted as "the human factor."

If you're planning a sexual adventure, you should also be creative. That doesn't mean you have to refurnish your apartment. This isn't a guide on interior design. I'm assuming that your apartment is furnished the way you want it. However, there are still some general rules that can be easily followed in order to bring a touch of eroticism into your apartment. A few accessories, placed and used accordingly, can turn an otherwise dull and repetitive evening into something more sustained and exciting. Taking charge of the situation is a challenge you have to accept if you want to make your sex life more interesting. If you already have a partner who is generally in charge, he will definitely enjoy some of your input. You'll find a few suggestions in the following chapters.

▼ Presented in the Right Light

The easiest way to vary a room's atmosphere is lighting. Dimming the lights, lighting candles—these are popular methods of creating a different mood. Screwing in a red bulb is slightly more daring, but its warm glow has set pulses a-racing in every brothel across the world. At least it makes everyone's skin look flushed with blood, which is generally flattering to most (half) naked bodies. The unfamiliar lighting will also heighten the other person's perception. Not just red lighting, blue or black lights also have a defamiliarizing effect. You can always find a lamp whose bulb can be easily changed in order to conjure up a different color. You can get suitable lamps and bulbs just about anywhere. While black light will have the effect of making your teeth and eyes look rather spooky—not to mention the glowing white bits of fluff that suddenly turn up everywhere—Osram's "violet" hue, when used on its own as the sole source of light will cast a mild, moonlike glow that makes everyone look good. My favorite, of course!

Changing the quality of the light during longer sessions is a useful method for refreshing the senses. After hours of action under the same unchanging light, there won't be much in the way of new sights. Turn up the lights, turn them down, light more candles, or fewer—it's easy enough to change the lighting. Total darkness will give you the opportunity to concentrate on other senses apart from sight (see *Master of the Senses*).

▼ Polishing up the Furnishings

Most of us tend to not have our own playroom at home where we can mess around to our heart's content. Of course, there's always the bedroom, but don't be afraid to incorporate your beloved living room, because that's where the comfort zone is generally a given. That's where you sip your drinks, listen to music, maybe watch a porno movie. And then: "Come on, let's go into the bedroom!" Such a pity! Enough of this misplaced respect for the civilized parlor, to hell with your fear of stains, throw yourselves onto the couch and screw each other silly!

If you have a passion for antique Chinese porcelain, you might want to keep your collection somewhere other than where you expect the action to take place. If you're constantly afraid of breaking something while you're having sex—for instance because you've placed a goldfish bowl on the glass table next to you—it's going to be difficult to relax and enjoy yourself. The same goes for mirrors, which I'll come back to later in the chapter *Master of the Senses: Through the Looking Glass,* and for wobbly furniture. You can probably have good sex on Chippendale chairs too, but if you want to disport yourself somewhere other than the bed or the floor, you need to at least offer a comfortable alternative. No matter what you decide on, whether it be a beanbag, an old flea-market stool, or an expensive designer chair, you can probably use the furnishings for all kinds of things. So, why not take that into account next time you visit the furniture store?

Aside from comfort or at least stability, your furniture's ability to cope with stains will also play a role. Good sex is dirty, in the physical sense too, and men tend to leak. From the back, from the front, pretty much everywhere. Of course, washable materials are a good choice, so it's best to go straight for leather or removable and washable upholstery. Otherwise, I'm still on the lookout for a cost-effective, flexible way of upcycling my less hard-wearing furniture into play equipment without completely disfiguring it. A thin vinyl cover, in black of course, is easily tailored—that should do it! You could use that to wrap up your couch and chairs without too much trouble and without them losing their attractiveness. After all, the

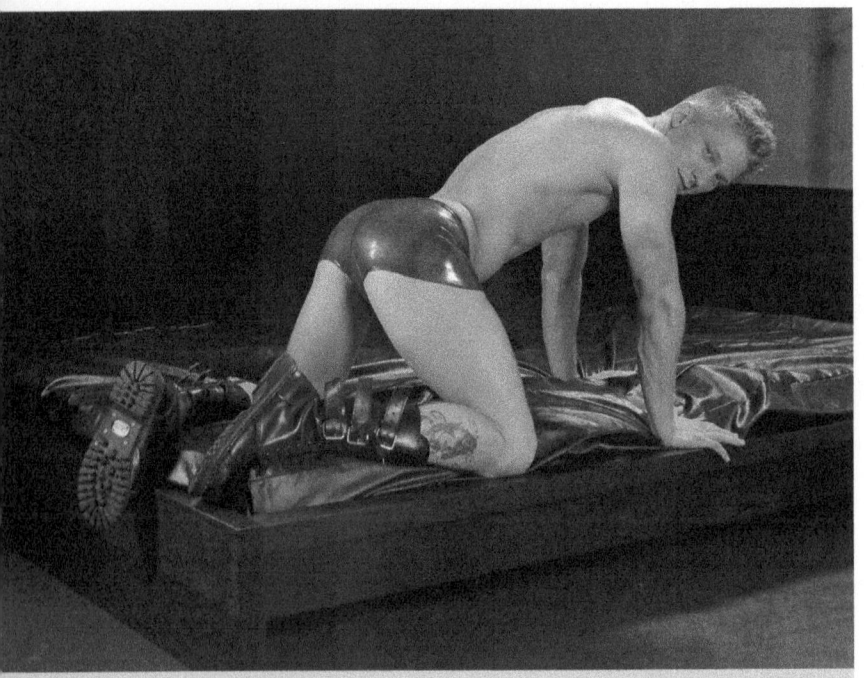

"How does my ass look in these shorts?"

plastic covers used by Fran Fine's mother in *The Nanny* are out of the question.

Large pieces of leather would be a better option, as they are pretty much indestructible. A cheaper alternative would be a pond liner, available from every hardware store in different styles and strengths. You can easily drape both of these options over everything standing around in the apartment, including the heirloom Persian rug, and voilà—your precious décor is now stain-resistant!

Furthermore, it is also water resistant. Which means that the water sports enthusiasts among us now have the opportunity to get going. You can save yourself the customary move to the bathroom. Not only can the piss or oil play commence with a light heart, you also don't need to worry about the consequences of conventional sex. It just goes to show how deep-seated our anxieties about our property really are when everything starts running smoothly all of a sudden on top of the slick material!

▼ **What's with All the Hooks on the Wall?**

Sex doesn't need to be an all-consuming presence in your apartment. After all, there are other priorities. Showcasing your dildos along with your best coffee cups will only distract your neighbor from your scintillating conversation, so just pop them in a drawer. On the other hand, if he happens to be cute and you want to go beyond drinking coffee with him, you might want to consider leaving them lying around somewhere in the open. Otherwise it shouldn't be hard to store these and similar utensils in an opaque container of your choice. Of course, you do need to consider your choice. A friend of mine's mother, having climbed the stairs to his apartment on the sixth floor, collapsed onto a stylish plastic object by Philippe Starck, taking it for a robust stool. The thing toppled over with his mother still on it, the lid fell open, and out rolled an assortment of dildos in all shapes and sizes.

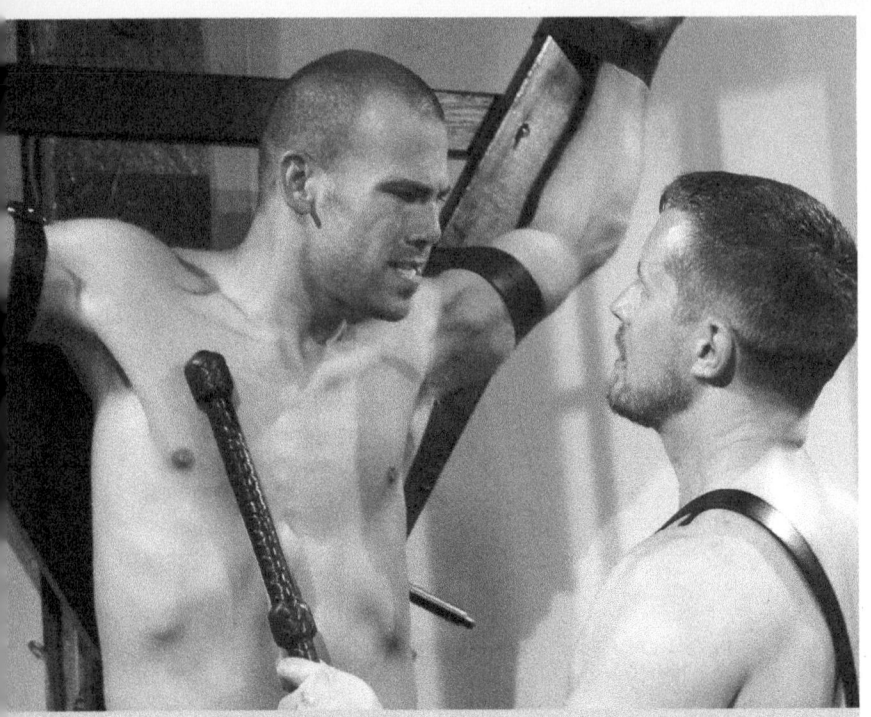

"Are you sure this is the kit for the Billy bookcase?"

It takes courage and practice to exhibit a certain amount of confidence when clear indications of your sexual practices are discovered. But, even when pertaining to other, less easily hidden equipment, it is also very sexy. Even a weight bench placed in front of a closet mirror can be used for other things than sports. Yet on the other hand, it's just a weight bench in front of the closet. *Honni soit qui mal y pense!*

Considering the popularity that slings enjoy in the gay community, they tend to be underrepresented in gay men's living rooms. If you believe the many testimonials on this subject, this is due to the "unsound walls," to "I don't know where to hang it," and "I don't feel like drilling holes!" Feeble excuses, all of them—where there's a will, there's way! So much energy and money is spent on built-in cupboards and wall ornaments, so why not find a way to hang up a sling? It might contribute a lot more towards improving your quality of life than yet another picture hanging on the wall.

You don't need to hang flower baskets off the wall hooks whenever the sling is not in use. (Although some concerned friends once gave me something similar shortly before my parents came to visit. But I didn't hang them up. That would have been even more suspicious!) I am sure you'll come up with a suitable answer, depending on who asks you what they're for. "I need them for my presentation!" or "I use them to attach partition screens to!" or "Do you really want to know?" served up with a nod and a wink. These are just a few suggestions. A couple of hooks or other fittings attached to the wall—available in all kinds of designs from hardware and furniture stores—are a great way to experiment and awaken your sense of play. The most important thing is to attach them properly, to a screwed-down bed or a steel plate if necessary, so as to distribute the pressure evenly. Attaching a couple of ropes and chains to the wall (and removing them again) should not pose a problem. Now you can try tying your partner to the wall. He will be securely fixed as long as the fixture can bear a greater weight than that of the guy you want to hang from it, without anything giving way.

When in doubt, or if you're still concerned about ruining your apartment, you need to find an alternative place to stay. How about renting a construction trailer for a short time?

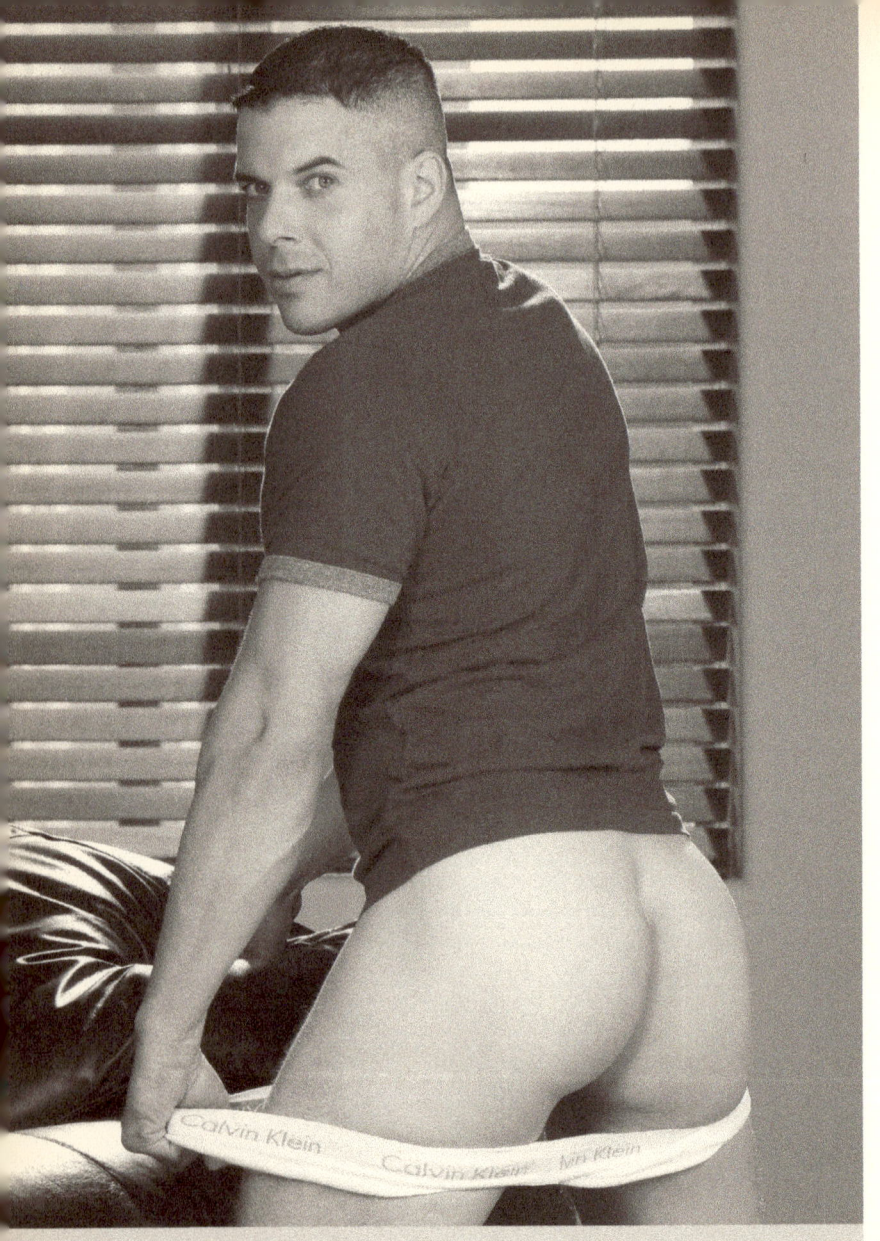

Being a good neighbor is all about sharing.

Rituals and Signals

"Custom is the enemy of desire"—you and your partner should have this motto embroidered on your pillow. Custom is habit, increased and multiplied until it reaches tedium. Habit, in the sense of familiarity, can be a positive thing. Being familiar with your partner, with his particular quirks, likes and dislikes, means you can be together without being stressed out—and this will only turn into a boring routine if you are led by laziness and thoughtlessness to go through the same motions over and over again. Truth be told: The more stress you have to deal with in everyday life, the more relaxing you'll find familiar, predictable sex, so please don't waste your strength on experimenting if you already expend more energy on the daily grind than you really want. In this case, doing the customary deed in a tried and true fashion can be a lot more beneficial. Rituals are there to make sex easier, as both partners can use signals to prepare themselves for what's about to happen. That doesn't mean that getting out the lube always has to lead to dropping your pants, but it *can* mean that, if that's the signal you've decided on.

This brings us to our first story, in which we'll make the acquaintance of the protagonists who will be accompanying us from now on. Brad and Corey are a couple who like to experiment and who are mainly interested in experiencing the physical intimacy of naked skin, while Bruce and Joaquin also use role-play and toys to get a psychological thrill out of the time they spend together. Both couples use signals in the proper sense. They act and react to certain looks, gestures and words, which serve to direct the course of the ensuing action.

Rituals and Signals—
First Softcore Sex Story with Brad and Corey

Before opening the drawer, Brad threw a cheerful glance at his boyfriend Corey, who lay on the bed in naked anticipation. Brad took the lube out of the drawer, leisurely placed it on the bedside table and laid a rubber down next to the bottle of slippery fun. He rubbed the plastic wrapping between his fingers, producing a rustling sound, and regaled Corey with a broad grin, reveling in the spectacle that presented itself on the white sheet. Corey's tanned body was sprawled in front of him as he began to stroke his chest and belly, then grabbed his hard dick and jerked himself off for a couple of slow strokes. This little show made Brad really horny. He let his cock jerk, to show Corey how turned on he was. A clear drop promptly appeared on the tip of his dick and remained hanging there, trembling, confirming his rising desire.

Now Brad watched as Corey's foreskin slipped over the smooth tip and then released it again as he jerked himself off. Corey put his hand to his mouth, spread his spit over his fingers and lubed his dick up with saliva until it shone wetly. *A gorgeous piece of ass!* Brad suddenly thought. His balls lay on the hairless thighs under the erect shaft and moved whenever Corey pressed his legs together hard in order to increase the hot feeling of suspense in his ass and dick. Brad approached the side of the bed with his pelvis thrust forward, his rod leading the way. The drop of pre-cum slid down his bobbing cock, barely missing Corey, who scooted over and, following his lover's directions, began to pamper his organ with his lips and mouth. Brad bent forwards and soon enough both of them were eagerly sucking and licking at each other's cocks, until they lay on top of each other, writhing and moaning lustfully on the bed. Corey's ass crack lay tantalizingly close as Brad worked his way down the shaft towards his balls. One flick of the tongue between his lover's plump cheeks, and immediately one leg wrapped itself around his shoulders, offering him a view of his anus. With the tip of his tongue he felt for the entrance to the warm soft interior, gently pushed open the ring of muscle, slipped inside and covered the delicate skin with saliva.

Oh man, that was delicious! A slap on his luscious ass made Corey turn over onto his belly, legs spread slightly to allow room for Brad, who threw himself on top of him and buried his face between his buttocks, noisily drawing his tongue down the crack, making the sensitive opening in the middle more and more pliable and willing. Brad shoved two fingers into Corey's mouth and enjoyed his sucking before pressing one, then two wet fingertips into his pliable anus. Corey made a growling noise and became more and more relaxed and ready for the other guy's dick. With considerable effort, he reached over to the bedside table for the wrapped condom and pushed it over the mattress towards Brad. Brad snorted in satisfaction—he liked it when Corey begged to get fucked. But this time he didn't feel like prolonging the foreplay. He grabbed the rubber, tore open the wrapping, rolled down the condom over his tool, and, supporting himself on both arms, penetrated the guy underneath him. He was so well prepared, they didn't even need lube; slick with bodily fluids, Brad gradually penetrated deeper and deeper until he was in up to the hilt.

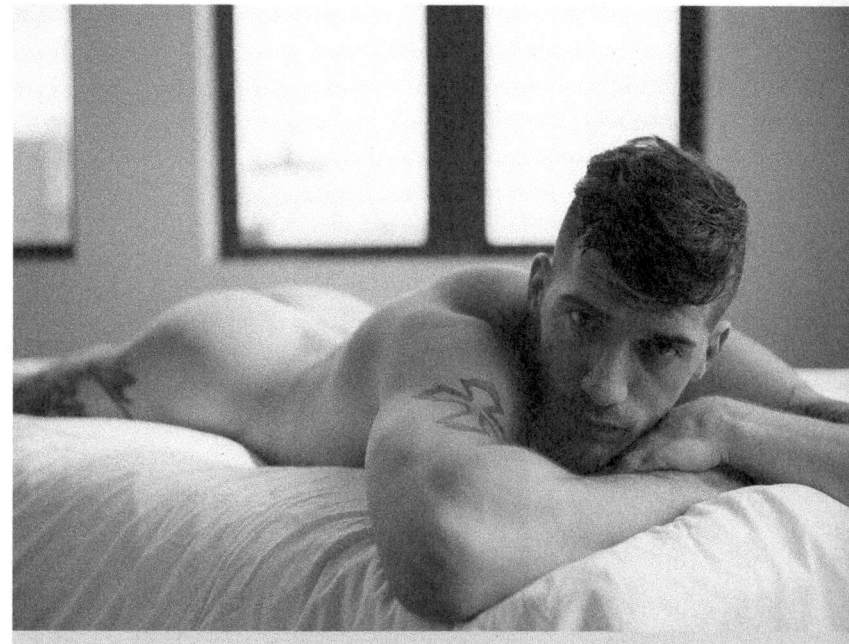

Corey's tanned body, for Brad's eyes only

The further proceedings could, according to taste, consist of an intense pounding, or a slow, concentrated in-and-out. There is not much to report on the copulation front, but fortunately the repertoire is already varied enough, thanks to the possibilities of changing orifices and positions. The beginning of the sex act between Brad and Corey should have been sufficient for the purpose of showing examples of rituals and signals. How many of them you will have noticed will depend largely on your own interpretation. In any event, Brad and Corey are a well-established team, able to use and extend the meanings of non-verbal signals. Perhaps they are seasoned pros who have paid attention and learned a lot during their countless adventures with other men, or perhaps they have found a way to clarify some of these signals. We will come back to the possible ways in which rituals and signals can be used and understood in a later chapter.

The world of S&M lovers is especially replete with signs and rituals. After all, tops and bottoms are sometimes called master and slave. The master gives the orders and the slave obeys. A certain amount of understanding for narrative is a necessary condition for this type of role-play, which can be completely choreographed like a play so that a certain cue or the appearance of a certain prop will start off the next move. In order to prevent the course of the action from unconsciously falling into a routine, the meaning of every cue must be clear to both partners. This ensures that they function independently of one another and are capable of sustaining suspense and arousal. Bruce and Joaquin will demonstrate this here. So, let us pay close attention to the first steps of their S&M play!

Rituals and Signals— First Hardcore Sex Story with Bruce and Joaquin

The doorbell rang precisely at 10:00 p.m. Bruce pushed the buzzer and left the apartment door ajar. He then retreated to the living room and leaned back comfortably in his TV recliner. He took a sip from his beer and leisurely continued to watch the porno movie. His anticipation hung heavy in his balls, which were nestled in their jockstrap, but he couldn't be bothered to achieve a full erection. After all, it was another man's job to take care of that! He heard Joaquin close the apartment door and knew that he was peeling off his clothes and would soon be putting on the fetish gear that Bruce had left lying out for him in the hallway. The black lycra ski mask covering his face from his mouth to his eyes would lend him a certain measure of anonymity that turned both of them on and made it easier for them to let themselves go. The jockstrap Joaquin was to wear wasn't the freshest and was already streaked with stains of piss and semen left over from their last date.

Bruce smiled to himself at the idea of Joaquin picking it up and briefly sniffing at it before putting it on. The used thing's smell gave him a feeling of cozy familiarity. Apart from the mask, the jockstrap, and his sneakers, Joaquin was now naked. Shortly afterwards he knocked at the door.

"Come in," Bruce called without turning round. He heard Joaquin approach and watched as he kneeled down in front of his spread legs, between the heavy leather boots.

"I'm glad you're here!" said Bruce to his toy boy as a greeting.

"I'm looking forward to you!" came the reply.

"Feel like getting dirty?" Bruce asked him. Not satisfied with the answering nod, he asked again "Do you?"

"Yes!" said Joaquin.

"Yes, what?" Bruce wouldn't let it go.

"Yes, I feel like getting dirty!" Joaquin finally replied.

But Bruce still wasn't satisfied. "For example?" he probed.

Hesitantly at first, but with increasing enthusiasm, Joaquin listed their customary activities. He wanted to lick Bruce everywhere, he wanted to be fucked by him, have his ass spanked by him. Bruce was satisfied. "It's up to you whether all of that will happen, is that clear?" Bruce explained brusquely.

Again, just a nod from Joaquin at first.

Bruce slapped him. "Is that clear?" he repeated.

Joaquin hastily affirmed his willingness. Yes, he would do anything for that to happen.

First of all, he had to fetch the leather handcuffs lying ready next to the recliner. Bruce grasped his right arm firmly, twisted it, and stared at it intently for a while before attaching the cuff. This was followed by the left arm, the left cuff.

With one hand, Bruce tapped the jockstrap between his legs. "Fetch me the crop!" he ordered. Joaquin brought him the thin, leather-bound riding crop with the flat leather flap at the tip. Bruce told Joaquin to present his entire body for inspection: his mouth, his ass, nipples, dick, balls. Joaquin had to show him everything and let himself be felt up. Bruce loved to contemplate another guy's genitals. He found them freshly intriguing every time. It gave

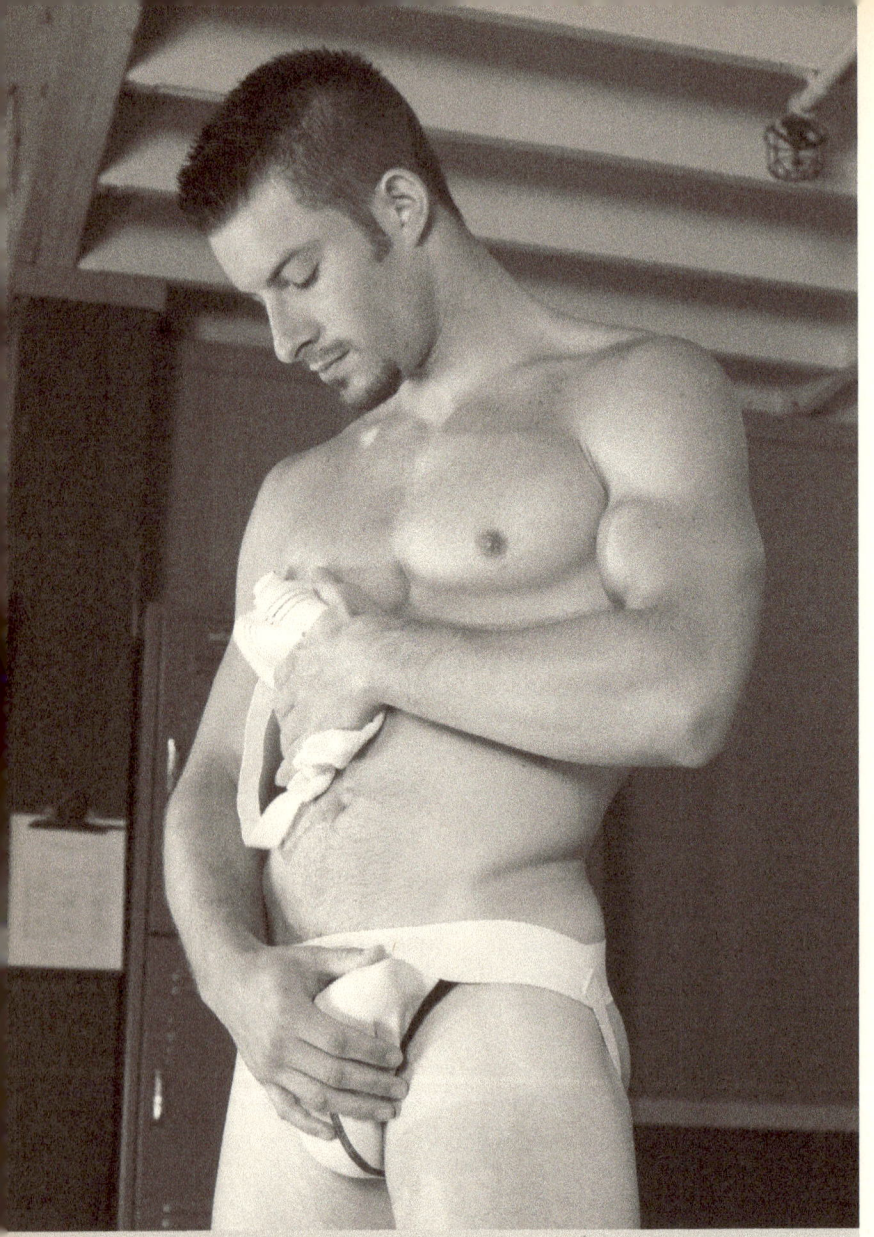

Bruce's anticipation hangs heavy in his balls.

him a real kick. A light touch with the riding crop was enough to let Joaquin know what part was up next. If he wasn't quick enough for Bruce, a quick blow got Joaquin going.

Eventually both of them ended up in the same position as before: Bruce on the recliner with Joaquin kneeling in front of him. With one hand, Bruce tapped the jockstrap between his legs. During the course of Joaquin's hot presentation, his cock had swollen to respectable proportions and was longing to be pampered.

Joaquin immediately pressed his face into the thick bulge, but he was moving too fast for Bruce. He shoved Joaquin back, grabbed his face and stared intently into the eyes that gazed at him through the holes in the mask.

"Not so fast, understand?" he cautioned Joaquin. "Nice and slow!"

Joaquin nodded, he understood.

▼ Sending Signals

The better the communication during sex, the more satisfying it will be for both partners. Showing what you like and what you don't like can be done in various ways. But even before embarking on a date with serious intentions, you can use a code to express certain sexual preferences, one example being the hanky code with its different colors, which has largely gone out of fashion. There is no need to boldly ask "Are you a top or a bottom?" if you send out signals that communicate this. In casual, witty conversation, you can make your intentions clear by using different phrasing ("I really like to fuck!"), unambiguous looks, gestures or touching—for example staring at the ass of the guy you've just met, licking your lips while smiling, or even laying your hand on his cheek.

Once you're aware of the meanings of individual signals, you can start to play with them. You can recognize them or use them for your own purposes. You can make them obvious or let them remain ambiguous. This requires concentrating on your partner. The better the dialogue between the two of you is, the more you can create closeness, giving you both the chance to instigate a sexual encounter that will be an intense experience for both of you.

▼ Words

Not exactly the easiest way of expressing something, but always worth a try: If you want something, *say so!* A certain amount of feeling for the right timing is part of it, too, but, when charmingly expressed, formulating a fantasy is usually welcome. If your fantasy is rejected, there are two possibilities:

You need precisely this fantasy in principle or simply right away in order to experience good sex. Then you'll presumably abort the entire thing. The problem with this type of specialization is, of course, that you are giving up the possibility of having satisfying sex with the guy you have chosen to be your partner in any other way.

If you're more flexible and willing to give the guy a chance, you need to tune in your sensory antennae and try and find a common denominator. Apart from the rejected fantasy there must be other things you can enjoy with him, if you like him in principle. Does he make any suggestions? Does he betray his erotic desires in other ways? Perhaps there will be another time, and your guy will come around to the fantasy he rejected before. Perhaps he'll show you his own fantasies and you might learn something, maybe even about yourself. Words can simply be an aid to clarifying what happens between you and your partner physically. This is the basis for good sex. Dirty words, simple words can be incredibly liberating, so why beat about the bush? "Turn around!" "Kneel down!" "Open your mouth!" Men love clear, unequivocal words and signals. Maybe this stems from their past as hunters, when there was no time for long explanations? Garnishing the directions with a tender pet name–"Turn round, honey!"–or with an insult–"Kneel down, you hot slut!"–is critical to successfully implementing your signal. If your partner is not used to your hurling abuse at him, a certain amount of caution is advised.

You can try feeling your way by using humor, for example a half-joking "You like that, you cocksucker!" You'll soon see whether your partner goes along with it or not.

I'm assuming that the object of your desire is in some way attractive and sexy or that there's at least something about him. If you want to experience real closeness, paying him an honest compliment won't kill you. That doesn't even have to get too personal. It's enough to celebrate the man-sex the two of you are currently enjoying in general, and to be conscious of experiencing this together. Instead of saying "Your cock is delicious!" you can express your enjoyment of sex by saying "Cocks are delicious!" and your partner will definitely understand the compliment being paid to him, not so much as a person but as an object of desire.

In S&M practices, ritualized forms of communication, verbal or otherwise, are employed. Certain commands demand a certain response for the action to continue. As a rule, the previously negotiated safe word that stops the action lies outside of normal communication, so that a "No, please!" can be a possible element of role-play. "Antidisestablishmentarianism" does fulfill these conditions, but the participants will generally come up with a better word. It is customary to repeatedly test the safe word during the session as a matter of routine ("What is the safe word?") without stopping the action, so as to ensure that the receptive partner will be able to recall it at the right moment.

Catchwords taken from porn should be used sparingly or not at all, but sometimes you might not be able to come up with anything other than "oh, that's so hot!" And if you really mean it, then why not? It's better to talk nonsense than to just lie there mutely like a lump on a log.

▼ Looks

The best! To be able to read someone's thoughts in their eyes, you need to be wearing the right glasses. In order to know the other person's desires, you have to want to understand him. Even then, further clarification by other means is necessary under certain circumstances, for example, you won't be able to tell his HIV status by looking into his eyes.

Making eye contact is a good way of increasing intimacy, overcoming your shyness of one another, and sending out signals in any sexual context. Holding another individual's gaze creates trust, we can see this quite clearly in the animal kingdom, for example, where the flight reflex and pack order are controlled by eye contact. Waiting for the other person's reaction while holding his gaze, or sending out a signal yourself, will heighten your sensitivity for the human interaction between you and your partner—it helps with the fine tuning. With a look, you can ask for his consent before you perform an action, or find out how he feels about it once you've already started. If you can tear your eyes away from his dick and sink your gaze into his, before your mouth gets to work on his cock, you can set off a firework display in both of your heads, making the customary practice of oral sex much more intense, as you suddenly realize what's happening and who it's happening with.

Smiling or winking can create a real quantum leap—the more sincerely you mean it, the more smoothly you can move on. Gazing earnestly into another man's eyes while showing neither aggression nor the impulse to flee, has a very beneficial effect.

When you're exchanging intimacies it can create a brotherly feeling and alleviate anxiety. If it's just a brief encounter with a man, it can be a trigger for good or bad sex. It doesn't have to be romantic love you sense radiating from his iris—it's enough to see his consent, allowing intimacy in a glance. These visual caresses—aren't they the spice in your sex cookie?

▼ Gestures

Human beings have developed a large repertoire of universal gestures, largely independent from culture and origin. There are hand movements expressing invitation, resistance, encouragement, and moderation that do not require knowledge of divers' signals or training as an air traffic controller. If you are aware of them and use them during sex you will be surprised at how well they work. Pay attention, and you will see that they are used and understood by couples more than you might have thought.

Unambiguous gestures can be very sexy without being vulgar. Words can sound unnecessarily harsh, using the gentler notes of gestures you may not be able to communicate as clearly, but it will be a lot easier.

You can also send out signals using body language. If you present your ass or your dick to your partner, you are unmistakably telling him to direct his attention to this or that body part. Other gestures are less direct and allow your partner more leeway as to how to interpret them and decide what to do with them, as long as you do not send further signals. This leaves some space between the two of you and you can approach each other gradually.

In S&M practices in particular, there are a number of submissive and dominant positions that follow a set ritual. If a man kneels on the ground with his arms behind his back and his mouth open, you can probably deduce the meaning yourself. It's up to your personal interpretation where playful desire stops and S&M begins. A slap on the ass doesn't necessarily have to be interpreted as the act of a sadist towards a masochist. Apart from how it feels on your skin, which we will come back to later, it can also be a signal for your partner to change positions.

Closing your eyes as a gesture of acceptance and trust is another noteworthy point. I was surprised to find that even old-fashioned hand kissing is popular in a sexual context. It is a gesture of respectful affection or gratitude, uniquely unambiguous and, in my opinion, a very fine thing, especially between two men, even if there is no ring glittering on a finger and demanding to be kissed.

▼ Laughter

There is nothing better than the refreshing laughter after hot, intense sex, when both partners, overcome with joyful pride and a touch of relief, let out the physical satisfaction of their dicks, their hearts, and their heads in a hearty laugh!

Only once have I ever experienced a similar laugh, when I did a short stint of fencing. At the time, I was astonished as the tension resolved after a thoroughly choreographed exercise, once the courtly bow had

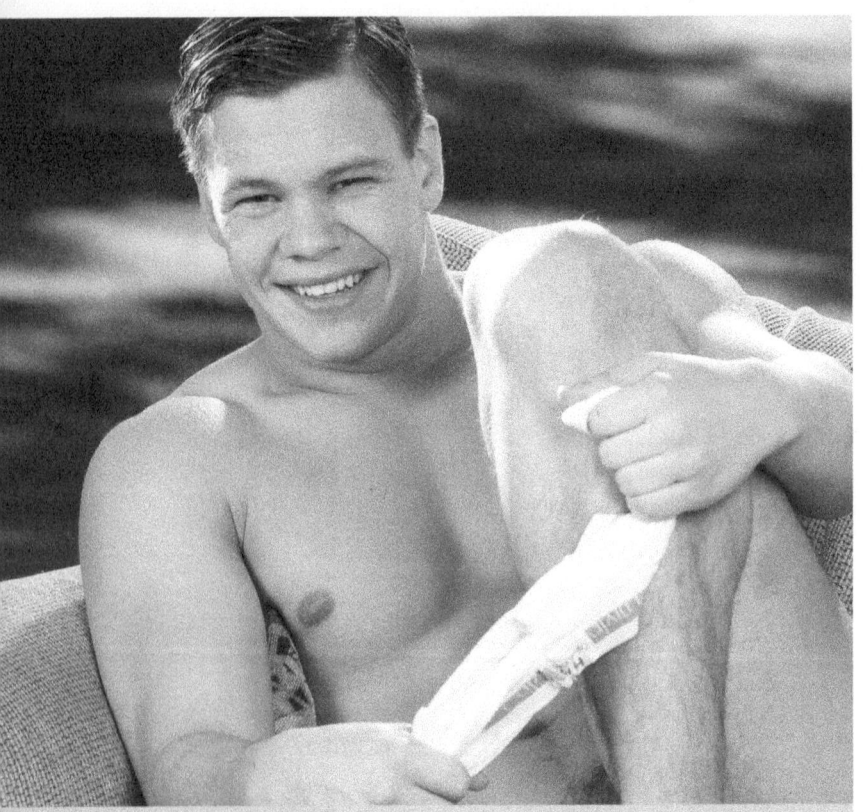

He's laughing with you, not at you.

been taken and my fencing partner and I finally tore the masks off our faces. We just had to laugh.

In the interests of our ground rule of respect, you might want to suppress the laughter that threatens to overcome you at the first sight of certain body parts of a previously unknown man—unless, of course, it's a happy, delighted laugh. Some men are also particular about their tattoos and piercings and won't appreciate your laughing at them.

Otherwise, good sex should be fun, and laughter is part of that—before, during, and after. Especially if something goes wrong, laughter can get you both back in the mood. That doesn't mean you should force it, but be open to it and let it out if you feel like it, and be pleased if your partner laughs. After all, it is and will always be an expression of happiness.

▼ Clothing

Having sex with a naked partner creates the best conditions for physical closeness. But because our brain has its own mysterious ways, other kinds of sexual stimuli are also possible, if certain items of clothing are used. A man can recall the associations another man's shoes, socks, underpants, pants, jacket, etc., have for him. Whether they evoke a traumatic experience or an erotic fantasy, both can be incorporated pleasurably into sex. People have such a close relationship with their clothes that I can't imagine a gay man not being able to develop an erotic relationship with any item of male clothing and then incorporating it into his sex life.

Why not try and see whether it will turn you and your partner on if you focus on, say, sneakers/underpants/socks, by simply wearing these and nothing else during sex. Apart from anything the sight of them might cause inside your head, there are other components that also play a role. More on this later in the chapter *Master of the Senses*.

Undressing a fully clothed man bit by bit or watching him take off one item of clothing after another creates a transition between distance and closeness, whose speed you can determine yourself, if you want to.

Of course, suddenly being confronted with the most intimate parts of another man—off the cuff, so to speak—when he remains clothed and, for example, just takes out his dick, or you do it for him, has its own special charm as well. This can only become a noteworthy occurrence if the appropriate glances have been exchanged first. Otherwise it's just another tasty cock-sausage on your list.

As a rule of thumb, you should always dress the same way as the object of your desire. So, if you want to land a skater, you need to dress like a skater, the same goes for leather, rubber, sportswear, a construction worker's gear, or fashion in general. This rule is, in my opinion, not applicable if you wish to broaden your horizons. The universe has a wide variety in store for us—but, of course, this corresponds to my personal, rather general preference: men!

On the other hand, uniformity can be a great way to experience gay sex, as it transforms its wearer into a universal hot idea and creates a feeling of affinity. Strict dress code parties are a great invention for this very reason. They offer you the chance to experience, for a limited period of time, the world outside of the everyday.

Certain types of clothing will influence your sexual behavior, whether consciously or unconsciously. If one partner is fully clothed during sex while the other is buck naked, this unusual constellation can create a special arousal curve. Sending your partner on ahead into the apartment and asking him to strip naked and lie, sit, or kneel on the bed or wherever, and then standing before him fully dressed can blow a new, surprisingly hot wind in the drooping sails of your sex life!

In the right circumstances, clothes can be a turn-on. Especially if you're choosing an outfit for your date—one that doesn't correspond to your everyday clothing and possibly only sees the light of day in a sexual context—the erotic effect will make itself felt not only by

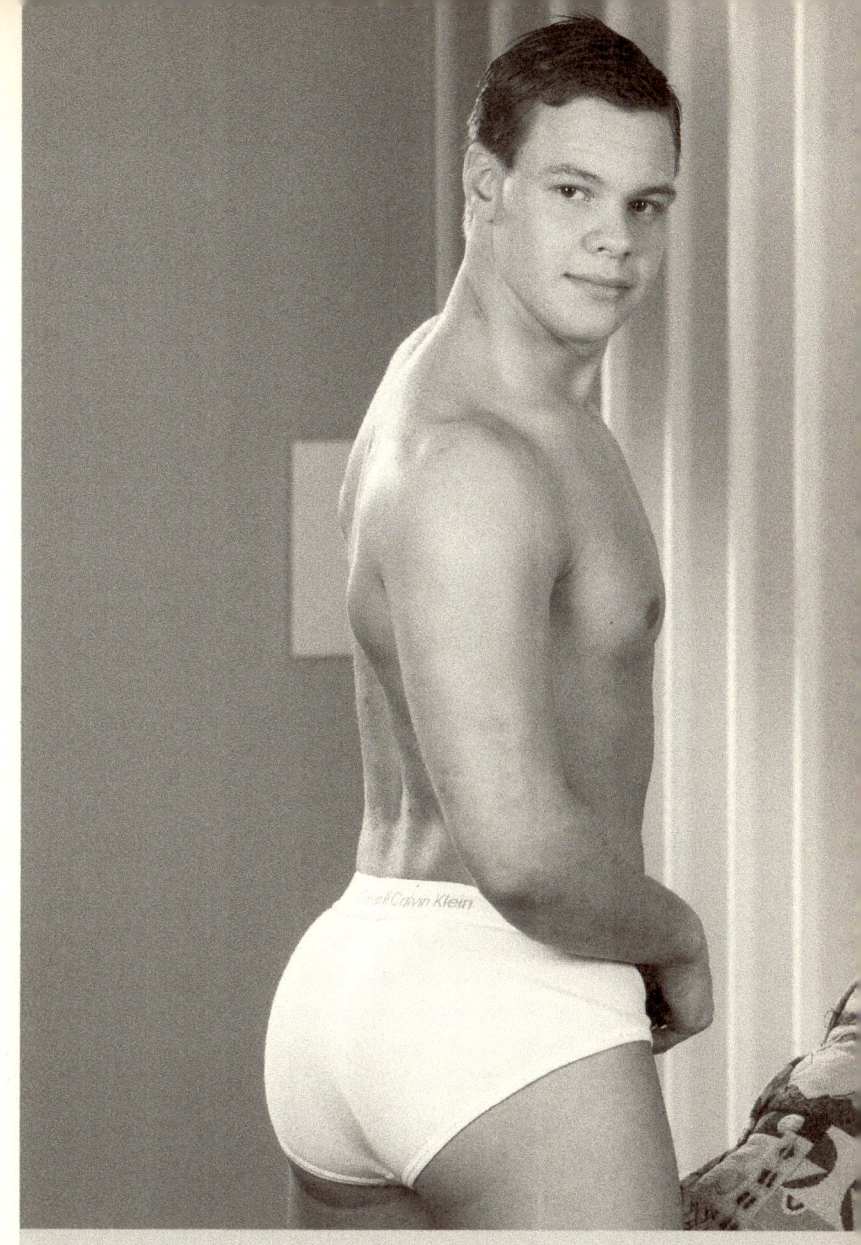

"Am I overdressed for this party?"

you, but in your surroundings. You will definitely stand differently in heavy boots than you would when barefoot or wearing sneakers, and you will walk out into the world differently. Leather or rubber on your naked skin, wearing jeans or sports pants without underpants—all of that can take you on a journey into a land of sexual adventure, perhaps even while trying them on at home. Really showing your preferences takes courage and passion, but none but the brave deserve the fair! A trip to a gay fetish store or a second hand store doesn't always have to end up with you buying yet another T-shirt. Maybe next time you'll try on a pair of leather pants or rubber boots?

The more comfortable you feel in the item of your choice, the sooner other people will go along with it, having discovered a common interest or perhaps because you have piqued their curiosity. There definitely has to be some kind of agreement as to clothing styles—after all, while a pair of cycling shorts may have a stimulating effect on one guy, it can be a complete turn-off for another.

Apropos of cycling shorts: The condition your clothes are in is also a factor in your sex life. Freshly laundered—or freshly shined shoes, gleaming with polish—or sweaty, dirty, and stained? Different conditions can have different effects, but that way, they can also lend a certain breadth to the game. Breaking your typical habit always helps to stave off boredom!

▼ Things

The proper accessories can round off the signals you send out, if you want. Only hardcore fans wear their sexual preferences in the open: a slave collar (unless you're a Goth), handcuffs (unless you're a police officer), a can of Crisco attached to your belt, nightsticks and cockrings on your leather jacket, etc. The times when a leather band worn on the left or right arm told you whether your partner was a top or a bottom are long gone. Current fashions have killed off this signal, as men of all ages are, thanks to H&M, all currently wearing these things without committing themselves in the slightest. The hankies

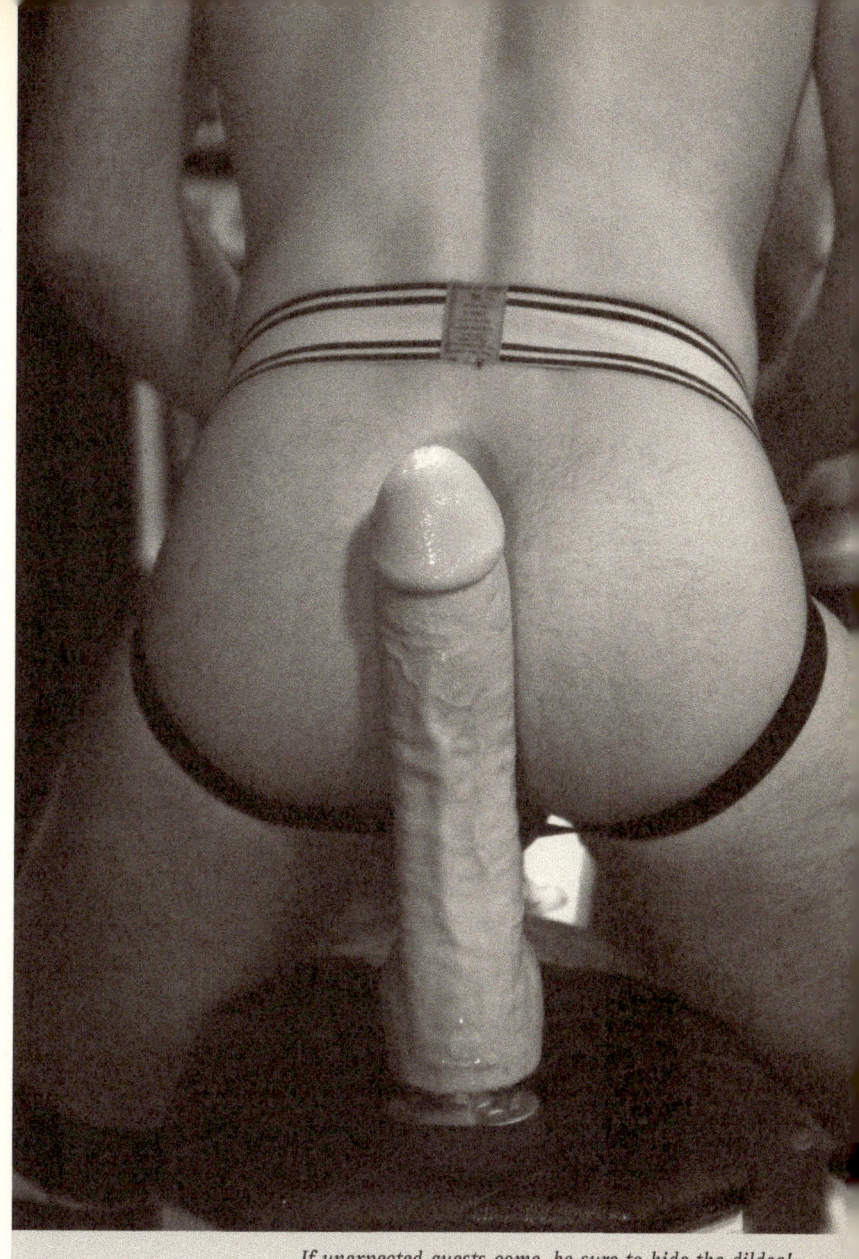

If unexpected guests come, be sure to hide the dildos!

or colored scarves that used to signify a top when worn on the left, and a bottom when worn on the right, have also gone out of fashion. Worn around the neck, they used to signalize both. At best, the color codes play a role in communicating personal preferences online.

Here is a brief overview of the most important color codes:

- pink - dildo play
- white - masturbation
- bright pink - toys
- light blue - blow jobs
- dark blue - fucking
- grey - bondage
- black - BDSM
- red - fisting
- yellow - piss play
- brown - scat
- khaki - military
- bright green - role-play
- orange - anything, anywhere, anytime
  (Just be careful, this may be taken at face value!)

As a rule, it's better to leave most of those accessories that can also be used as toys at home. They can always come into play as a nice surprise, and every well-appointed gay household should included a certain number of them. In our chapter *Master of the Senses*, we will be discussing some of them, but your friendly sex shop adviser should be able to show you a few things that will pique your curiosity as to what you could do with them and how your partner might react. Discovering each other with these aids can create intimacy, which is one of the most important requirements for good sex. These aids can either be offered to your partner from the outset or produced later at the appropriate juncture, depending to how you wish to present them. A newly purchased bottle of lube or massage oil can be a gift you can both enjoy, just as much as a dildo, a leather flogger, or something from the medical department, a speculum, a catheter, or similar equipment.

Sex in Clothing—Second Hardcore Sex Story with Bruce and Joaquin

On his knees, Joaquin slowly approached the jockstrap and the bulge it concealed. He saw how it outlined the contours of Bruce's semi-erect dick and discerned the tip of it on the left side of Bruce's loins. The fabric's original white coloring had given way in places to a grubby grey with yellowish brown edges. Joaquin could smell a faint tinge of piss, a biting smell of ammonia that went straight to his head and seemed to tickle part of his brain. Joaquin breathed deeply and the tingling sensation spread to other parts of him. Then the dick began to pulsate underneath the fabric. To be on the safe side, Joaquin looked up and met Bruce's tense gaze and an encouraging nod. With something akin to relief, Joaquin buried his face in the bulge between his boyfriend's legs, breathed in his scent, and tried to stick his tongue under the waistband of his jockstrap to reach the naked skin of his cock and balls.

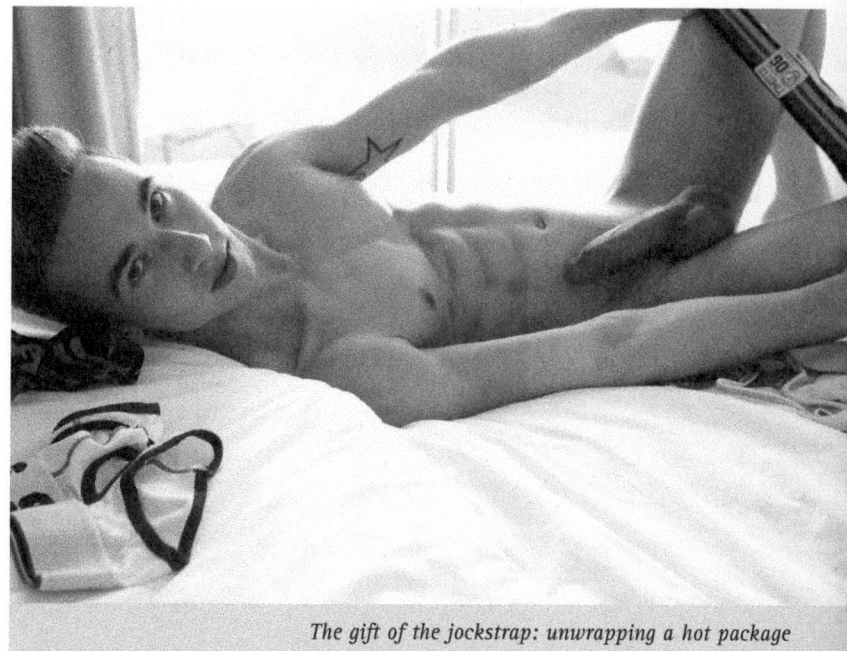

The gift of the jockstrap: unwrapping a hot package

Whenever his hands moved up Bruce's calves, over his thighs up to the jockstrap, Bruce slapped them away. He wanted to feel only Joaquin's mouth!

Once Joaquin's lips were nuzzling the place where the erectile tissue was, he felt the heat rise up from it and a fresh damp spot appeared on the fabric before his eyes. Like a wolf at a salt lick, he lapped at it, trying to get some of the delicious pre-cum onto his tongue. The greedy desire to see Bruce's dick and taste it grew stronger. Again, his hands crept upwards and onwards.

"Hands on my boots!" Bruce ordered curtly. Joaquin placed one hand on the left, the other on the right boot shaft and grasped the thick leather. This brought home to him the fact that his face was stuck right between another guy's legs, right on top of his bulging cock!

Again, Joaquin nibbled and licked at the jockstrap and with his teeth attempted to pull away the fabric and expose Bruce's dick. "Back!" Bruce commanded. Joaquin drew back and raised his upper body so that Bruce could get up and stand in front of him. Before his eyes, Bruce drew his nut sac out of the jockstrap and let it hang free. The little black hairs on the thick balls shone in the light as if they had been oiled. The things bulged out obscenely next to the fabric, which was incredibly hot! Joaquin approached them with his mouth open and looked at Bruce imploringly. He wanted to lap at them!

"Start at the bottom!" said Bruce.

Joaquin knew what that meant. He had to rein in his hunger and turn to Bruce's boots first. He kissed one, then the other in turn and licked the smooth leather. His hands closed their grip behind the boot heels. Bruce just stood there. Joaquin could feel the firm stance of his legs on the floor, making him feel more secure. Bruce was, in fact, just standing there, but somehow he was also floating. Conscious of keeping Joaquin's lust in check, feeling his longing to finally be able to reach his dick, the gentle throbbing of his mouth and tongue through the leather boots—all of this increased his anticipation for the moment when Joaquin's soft lips would encase his dick, which felt increasingly thicker and heavier. Of their own accord, his hands moved up and over his chest. He closed his eyes. Slowly, Joaquin worked his way up to the place where the sturdy legs emerged from the boot shafts. He kissed and licked the place where leather met skin—the kneecap, the knee—pressed a few gentle kisses onto the back of the smooth muscular calf, briefly lapped at the back of the knee and felt a shiver go through Bruce's skin. Upon seeing Bruce stimulating his nipples with his eyes closed, he let go of the boots and let his hands glide up Bruce's body, up his legs, unable to pass his naked ass cheeks without giving them a quick squeeze, up his belly to his chest. Bruce released his nipples and Joaquin pressed them gently with his fingers. Bruce moaned languorously.

Joaquin seized the opportunity and licked at Bruce's hairy legs in the immediate area around the jockstrap until he was finally able to once again press his mouth and nose into the hot package. While he was licking Bruce's legs, the face mask heightened the sensation of skin and skin, further arousing him. But he was only marginally interested in the jockstrap—he wanted to taste Bruce naked! He grunted in arousal into the fabric, his lust urging him on to more action. Hearing the demanding noises, Bruce's thoughts slowly turned back to Joaquin. Joaquin wanted more? Then more he should have! Bruce slowly turned his body to the left, allowing the other man's tongue to lick over the other side of his thigh, the elastic waist of the jockstrap, and over his ass cheek. Then he cried "Stop!" after which Joaquin ceased immediately and raised his upper body upright.

His eyes glinted through the holes in the mask, burning with anticipation of what would happen next. Bruce took a step away and bent his knees slightly. One glance back over his shoulder told him that Joaquin was waiting obediently while staring at the ass in front of him as if hypnotized. Joaquin was face to face with a muscular package framed by two elastic straps—two full and manly ass cheeks, with that incredibly sensitive and secret hole in the crack between them! Bruce reached back and pulled his cheeks apart to show Joaquin his anus, but only briefly, like a promise. Then he stood upright, bent his knees again in front of Joaquin's face, and held out his ass to him again. "Just the lips!" came the new order from Bruce. He luxuriated in Joaquin's soft kisses on his backside, slowly getting closer to the middle. He grabbed his cheeks again and presented Joaquin his hole. "Tongue!" was all Bruce said. Immediately, Joaquin touched the rim of his anus with the tip of his tongue, licked at it, and then ventured into the opening. With small thrusts, he dabbed into the soft tissue. Bruce groaned, let his hole twitch, and pushed out his ass further back, towards the incredibly hot feeling. Joaquin gathered up steam and licked and grunted at the crack to his heart's content! In the middle of this, Bruce took his hard cock out of the jockstrap and bent it back. Joaquin licked enthusiastically at the

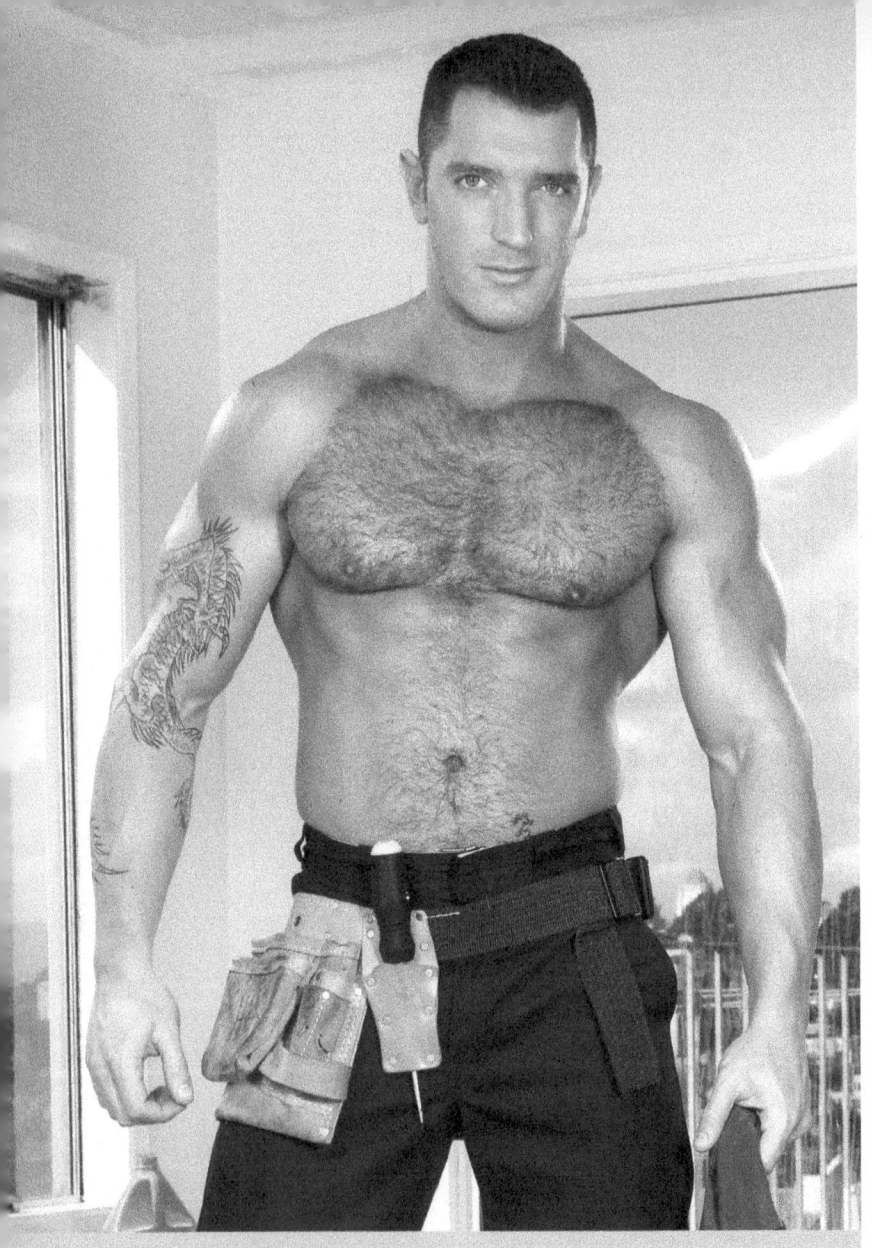

"No, I have not forgotten the hammer!"

juicy tip, but then the dick was jerked out of his reach once again and he turned back to his boyfriend's asshole.

Again, the knob returned to his mouth, Joaquin pushed his lips over the fat mushroom and sucked hard at the shaft. It felt great, the way Joaquin was sucking at his schlong, so Bruce turned around and pushed the whole thing into Joaquin's mouth up to the hilt. He pressed Joaquin's face into the stained jockstrap and stuffed his fuck rod down into his gurgling throat, feeling how the tip of it stimulated the tube of muscle. Saliva flowed out of Joaquin's wide open mouth. He choked on the thick wang. Swallowing his gag reflex, he felt the resistance of the tip opening up his throat. Wasn't that exactly what he had wanted, to have the whole thick cock pushed right in? Great!

Bruce pulled Joaquin's head back. His thick cock gleamed wetly as he drew it out of the greedy mouth. He stuck three fingers between the open lips, pressed down the tongue and pushed down. His gaze pierced the eyes that glittered at him from the holes in the mask.

Joaquin held his gaze, breathing steadily through his nose as he sucked at his fingers. He heard Bruce noisily drawing spit and then watched as a foaming wad of it formed at his lips and then detached itself. It plopped into his wide open mouth. Then the thick cock was pushed into his well-lu-bricated mouth again. Hungrily, Joaquin sucked at the chunk of manhood.

Master of the Senses

The main pleasure of sex is stimulating the senses. This sounds trivial enough, but with all the sensory overload we are subjected to daily, you are going to have to use extraordinary means to bring this pleasure to the fore! All five senses—sight, smell, hearing, taste, and touch—can be cranked up or soothed individually, turned on or off, or be alternately stimulated a little, a lot, or all together as part of a full-body experience. In general, unfamiliar stimuli have a greater effect than familiar ones, and a strong stimulus will leave a greater imprint on your consciousness than a weak one.

A man's body is a fantastic thing! Fat, thin, hairy, smooth—each one is a fascinating thing of wonder. Look at him, feel him, taste him and keep your nose and your ears open, so that you can smell him and hear him, too! This happens anyway during any type of sex, but usually not consciously enough. But it still stimulates us, it stirs up our subconscious. If you're up for great sex, you should turn your unconscious sensations into conscious enjoyment. By raising the stimulus threshold—for example through defamiliarization—you will be better able to understand your senses. That way, experiencing stimulation takes more concentration and will leave a more lasting impression. In the following pages, we will try out how to devote yourself to each of your five senses for a time. As our attention is limited—this will generally be sufficient to enhance your sexual experience—it isn't necessary to go through the entire repertoire and arouse each of the five senses individually or all at once. Touch and sight are the two senses that can be playfully influenced unobtrusively and with the most ease during the sexual act. Let's start with sight.

▼ The Eye of the Beholder

Men are triggered by visual cues. This phenomenon is the basis of all advertising. Even without sex, the right images are enough—and right away, part of brain, the hypothalamus, starts to secrete a hormone that increases the production of testosterone and thereby sexual arousal. The constant presence of stimulating images in porn, sex magazines, and online has raised our stimulus threshold so that we don't go about with a permanent hard-on. That's why putting on a porno DVD is not the most effective way of cranking up the mood, but it is certainly the most widespread. That is, of course, totally legitimate—after all, we are all susceptible to a hot sight, even if it is consumption, pure and simple. But if you want to play around with your sense of sight or occasionally cut it out completely, you will have to turn to other means.

Seeing is dependent on light. The less light there is, the less the eye is able to do its job of receiving visual stimuli. It has to work harder to see anything in the dark or semi-darkness. This heightens your concentration on what you see. Every halfway interesting darkroom works with the interplay of light and darkness, as the change also has a stimulating effect on our emotional brain, the limbic system, the seat of our emotional drives. What happens when the room you're in is totally dark because every source of light has been turned off or because the light is directly kept away from your eyes, with a blindfold for example? In the latter case in particular, your eyes are given a rest!

We have already described the gradations that are possible, up until total darkness, as well as the different light qualities (see *Presented in the Right Light*). Defamiliarizing effects such as colored lights or mirrors are particularly suited to changing the way you see things. The stimuli perceived in a new way create a more distinct and conscious impression. They are more difficult to store, but that means they stay in your head for a longer time. If you shift your concentration towards the visual experience, the other senses can take a break.

Shadow Play—Second Softcore Sex Story with Brad and Corey

Brad stood facing the wall while Corey remained seated on the chair, still panting with arousal from the intense mouth-fuck Brad had just treated him to. Brad stretched out his hand and switched off the overhead lights. For a brief time the room was plunged into total darkness, until Brad found the switch to the small halogen spotlight that lighted the mixer console. Lights up! He turned the struts around and twisted the globe at the head of the lamp so that the beam of light was focused between his legs. Brad moved his lower body directly into the light. His cock and balls gleamed brightly in the darkness, on stage like the main actor in a play. Corey watched in anticipation as he closed his hand around the shaft. In slow motion, Brad pushed the foreskin up, milking his dick until a shining drop of pre-cum oozed out of the slit. With the index finger of his other hand he played with the sticky fluid, a viscous cord stretching from his finger to the glans, until it finally dripped onto the floor.

His fingers slid downwards, raised his balls, enfolding them, squeezing the sensitive globes until the skin of his scrotum was stretched tight. A wad of spit landed on his shaved nuts, was spread around and made them shine. Corey was dying to lick them! On the other hand, he was loving the little show, enjoying the almost scientific look at his lover's most intimate parts, only a few feet away from him, within reach. Now Brad was beating off with slow strokes. His attention turned to the shadows, his movements created on the wall next to him. The angle of the light made the act appear larger—it looked like a black giant flogging his enormous hog!

When Brad looked back down at himself, Corey's illuminated face was floating in front of his dick, his gaze fixed trance-like on the fat glans, which glowed in the darkness, wet and red like a ripe fruit. Now his lover's soft lips closed over the sensitive tissue. Oh, that was so good! Brad closed his eyes and let himself be pampered ...

▷ Through the Looking Glass

A good way of rediscovering familiar images is to use mirrors. It might take a bit of courage to watch yourself in the mirror during sex, but men are born voyeurs, that's just the way it is, and the distance that a look in the mirror creates can fire up this preference. You watch yourself as if you were in a movie. As you generally only look at your face and maybe your upper body in the mirror during your morning shave, an all-encompassing look at the rest of your body in the mirror can be full of surprises. Seeing your partner through the looking glass is just as exciting. The coolly reflected image will reveal everything that happens, without shame or mercy, and that can be very arousing, it's like watching a live porno movie. Your intentions will be more or less apparent, depending on where you place the mirror. Of course, it's up to your partner, whether he

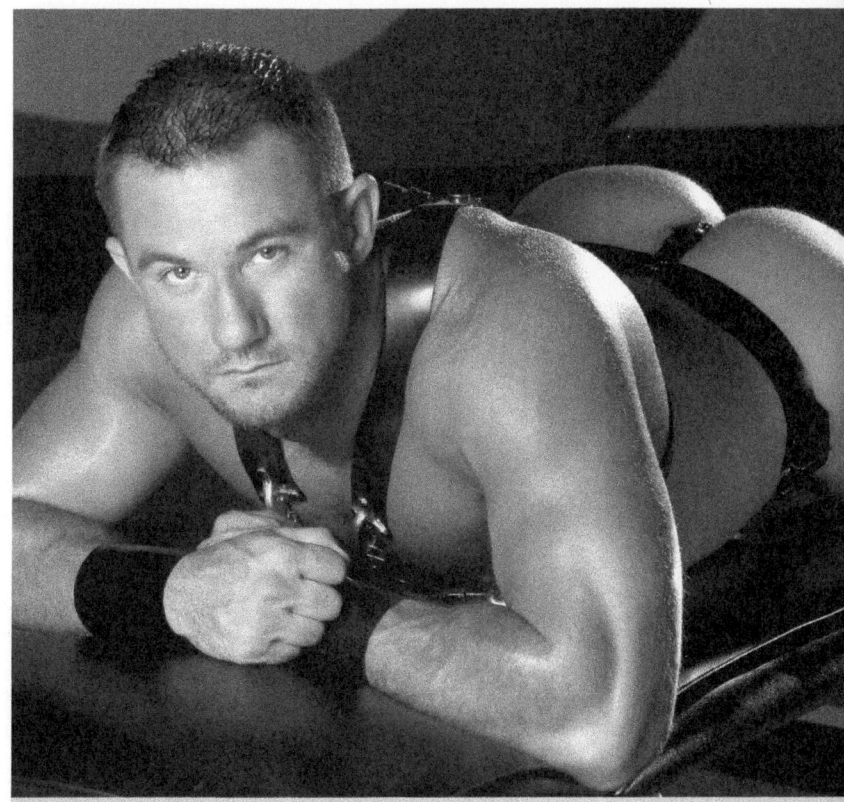

Looking cool, ready for the heat

joins you in watching through the mirror, or whether he prefers to look away.

Apart from the widely used wardrobe mirror, movable mirrors can be useful. For example, a pivoting mirror with a stand that you can both go to town under, or a simple framed or frameless mirror that you can place wherever you like. For the more intense or clumsy lovers amongst us I would recommend an aluminum mirror, for these are unbreakable. For a time I used to have a mirror as big as a door, which I would courageously place here and there, lengthwise or horizontally, but after the third mirror shattered—without causing too much damage, thank goodness—I had to start looking around for alternatives, not least because of the amount a mirror that size costs. You can find affordable versions at flea markets, for example. While you're there, you can also have a look at magnifying mirrors or concave mirrors. Set up at the right angle, these can be a revelation. Of course, this requires a refined technique with proper forethought as to how to fix and adjust your mirror, so as to avoid constantly having to readjust the thing and always needing a free hand.

Colored mirrors can also provide a welcome change. My personal favorite: blue glass!

A modern application of porno-vision is to relay the act to a screen via a camera. This allows for greater flexibility and the zoom will take over the function of a magnifying mirror without too many complications. Furthermore, you might have the option of viewing the action again at a later junction. This is a distinct advantage, but you should always remember that digital images have become part of our customary experience and are used over-extensively. Your own porno movie will drown in the sea of images that floods our over-taxed senses day by day. Shouldn't we give our sense of sight an occasional break, turn it off for a short time, not to sleep, but rather to use our other senses to experience an encounter with another man?

▷ Seeing the Light

Covering our partner's eye or both eyes with our hands is easy enough, and finding a piece of fabric to use as a blindfold should present no problem. From professional leather blindfolds and hankies to items of clothing, all kinds of things can be repurposed as a blindfold. The important thing is that they fit properly. Then you will know whether or not to continue. Once you've clarified that, you can downright celebrate putting on the blindfold. Before you tie it, you can present it, demonstrating its properties on other parts of the body or making your partner aware of its function by putting it on playfully. If that's too much for you, then just put it on yourself if necessary.

The blind partner is delivered from the constant stream of images and can concentrate better on his other senses and his own thoughts. Depending on what material you are using, light can still reach the retina. The light of a candle, for instance, waved back and forth before his blindfolded eyes, its light falling faintly through the blindfold, can be a precursor to wax play. It increases anticipation without an actual visual image. This works even better if you add acoustic signals. A riding crop whistling through the air, a condom wrapping being torn open—every sound is perceived and interpreted with heightened attention.

By taking away his sight, your partner's actions are greatly limited, making him more dependent on your attention and your actions. He has to wait for cues, which you can use to increase and extend the suspense. If you just feel like having comfortable sex, you can just lie down like a buffet and let him go on a discovery tour around your body.

If you would rather take the active part, there are loads of surprises you can come up with for the other senses—sex toys for touch or deliberately made noises for hearing, for these senses are now more responsive. But that isn't strictly necessary. Your body, taken inch by inch, is plenty interesting! No matter how and where you do it, if

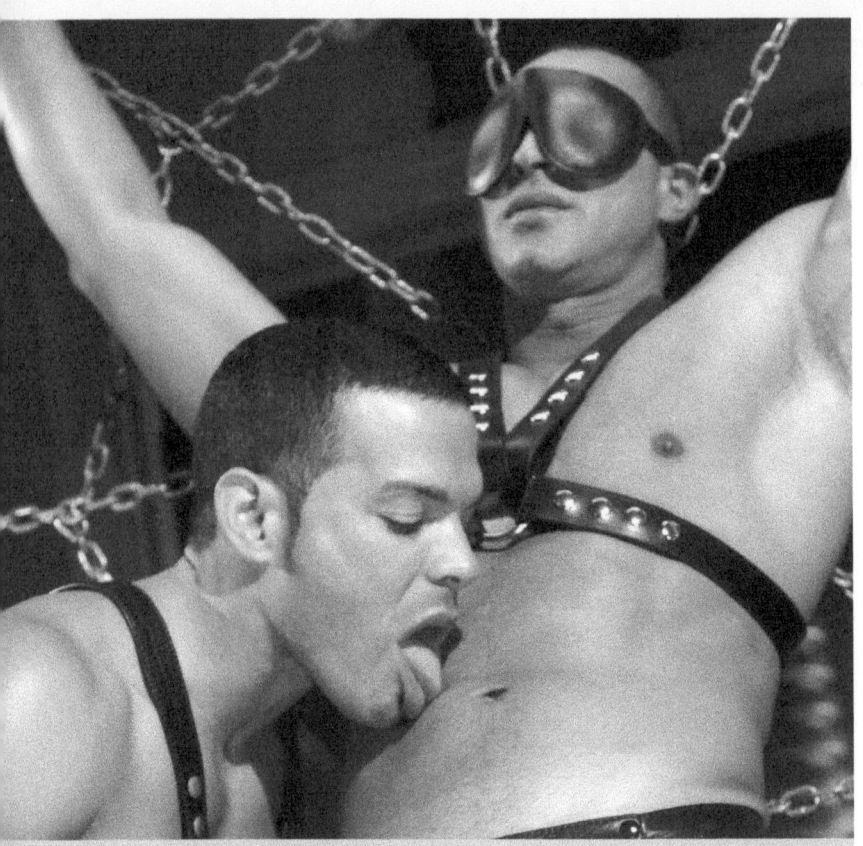

"I feel something wet ..."

you block out his sight, your partner can start to discover you anew. By commenting aloud on your actions, you can direct his attention, but you can do that without using words, with other signals—for example by simply leading his body.

While the blindfold prevents your partner from being aware of your gaze—no matter where you look, he has to put up with it—you yourself are completely protected. However bright the lighting is, it won't matter to you, you can be completely uninhibited. This is extremely relaxing and it also creates a power gradient, turning your partner into a delightful object, if that's the game you both want to play. Noiseless and secret acts should however be used sparingly, otherwise you run the risk of boring your partner. Hasty acts should not happen at all, these are unsettling and will spoil his enjoyment of being robbed of one of his senses. If an accident does happen, it's not enough to just laugh it off, you should also describe what went wrong. That way, he can understand what happened or adapt himself to the new situation. But aren't we all watching our own, completely private movie whenever we close our eyes, when we can only hear, smell, and feel?

▼ A Touch of Passion

With regard to the sense of touch, every body is unique. The size and variety of the organ in charge of this sense—your skin—explains its significance, but your skin's individual constitution is the basis of your own personal sense of touch. Skin has several layers, and its thickness and consistency varies from person to person as well as according to the parts of your body. Whether you find a sensation painful or enjoyable can vary widely. A man's nipples are a very good example, these being a regular feature of gay sex life. You can hang a small car from some of them without giving rise to much more than a weary yawn, while others you can barely touch without eliciting an agonized scream. This can even vary with the same man, depending on what mood or what stage of arousal you happen to catch him in. This varying sensitivity alone is enough to justify their existence—may they always remain a mystery in every other respect.

The sensations felt via the skin cover an almost infinite spectrum. The slightest breeze can, in the right circumstances, have astonishing results. Blowing, nibbling, biting, tickling, stroking, rubbing, squeezing, pressing, pinching, pulling, tapping, hitting, poking, and pricking are only a few examples. In addition, you've got the amount of pressure behind the stimulus, but moisture and dryness, heat and cold, also create special sensations on your skin.

The greatest density of receptors for tactile sensations can be found in the tongue, the erogenous zones and the fingertips. Let's say your partner is leading your hands—do you think you could correctly identify parts of his body by touch alone, even with your eyes closed?

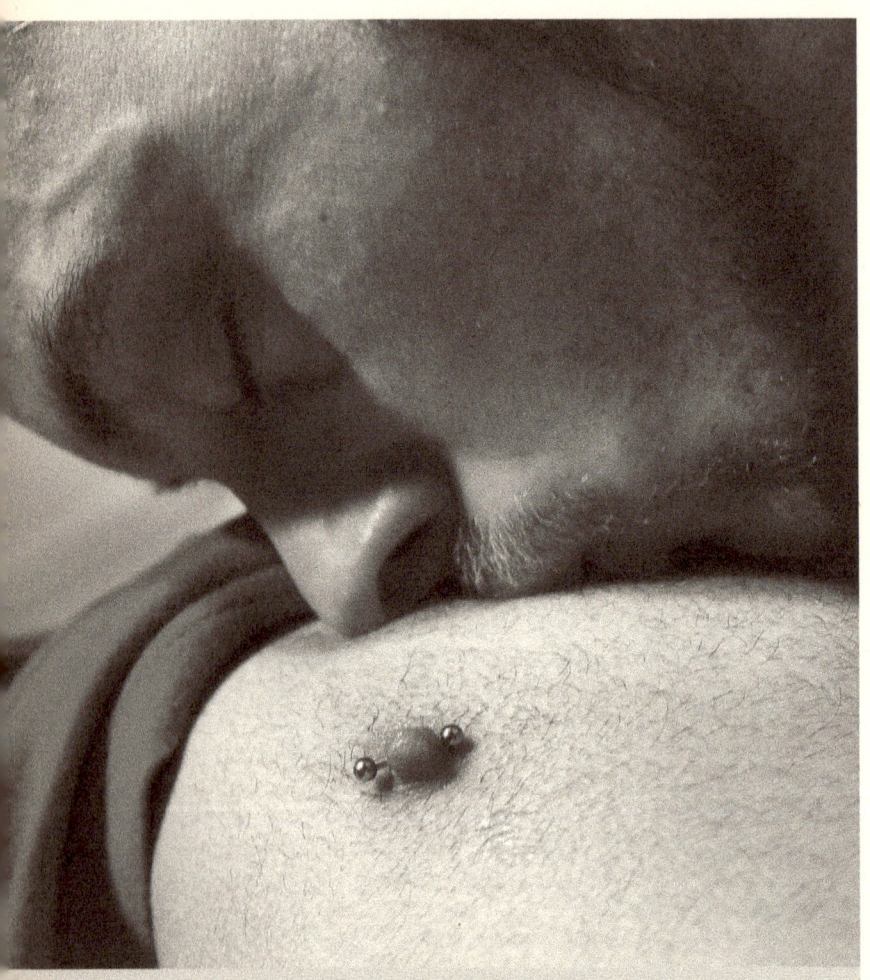

The tongue searches for the nipple.

▷ Scratch Me, Bite Me!

Apart from the fingertips, the mucous membranes are the most receptive to tactile sensations, but every part of your body can be stimulated and made to play the main part. The realm of touch extends from your toes to the crown of your head, but there is no limit to your creativity regarding other aids you can use. Even a piece of toilet paper held in your fingers can turn pinching and twisting into a new experience, while clingfoil or aluminum foil will transform the impression even more. You can find both of the latter in a pack of cigarettes, which can be turned into a little toy box. Gentle aids, such as feathers or fur, or rougher ones like brushes and sand, can be used as well, as can wet ones, dry ones, hot, or cold. For a longer, more intense session, an ice cube, applied at the right moment, can cause a wonderful reawakening of the over-taxed senses, especially if it comes into contact with the sensitive mucous membranes or even placed inside an orifice.

I don't need to tell you that a comfortable temperature should be a given for sex. It will be more difficult for you to pay attention to the finer sensations of touch if you're cold. However, localized fluctuations of heat and cold—for instance, when using ice cubes—are delightfully exciting. Besides ice, alcohol also has a cooling effect—you can get handy disinfectant wipes at the drugstore, for example.

If you want to use heat to stimulate the skin, you can warm up any household oil. Adding cinnamon, pepper, or chilies to the oil first will give it an extra kick. These are listed in order of pungency, which is translated to heat on your skin. Even toothpaste, smeared on the nipples or the glans, can, thanks to its menthol content, have an unusual but definitely stimulating effect. But it's not really a favorite, not least because the smell automatically evokes associations of dental care.

A heat rub to increase circulation, such as IcyHot, can warm up the blood and create a proper rush of heat. It can be dabbed carefully onto the nipples using a Q-tip, for example. After some time, the area will become very warm. Be sure to avoid getting the ointment in your eyes or on any mucous membranes! It's best to try it out on yourself first so that you can gauge the effect.

Sharp instruments such as razor blades and knives, or pointy ones such as needles and nails, are the province of S&M and should be treated with care. Hot wax falls under the same heading, but is always worth a try in my opinion. Store bought candle wax is not as hot as you would generally think, and it is easy to regulate the dose. A rule of thumb: the further away the candle from your body, the more time the wax has to cool down before it touches the skin. Beeswax on the other hand is not suitable as it gets too hot! I would always recommend trying it out on the back of your own hand before you start messing about with dripping wax.

Even without aids, your hands and mouth will provide you with enough possibilities to deliberately accentuate parts of your partner's body by concentrating only on these parts—or you can pamper his entire body from top to bottom, for example, with a massage.

One special form of stimulation is the use of an electric massage unit, also called an e-stim unit. The safest option is to buy a unit from a sex shop or an electronics store. If the two of you are using it, the procedure is approximately as follows: You hook it up to a piercing or a metal cock ring, turn it on, and your partner becomes the positive pole and you're the negative pole, or vice versa. Combined with moisture or mucous, such as a tongue or a nipple, the voltage is discharged with a perceptible tingling sensation or with a whipping blow, depending on how the input is. Other possible contact points between mucous membranes are self-explanatory. It is absolutely essential that you take care when gradually raising the voltage intensity and the impulse frequency. An interest in experimentation is required, but it is relatively safe as long as you don't hook up anyone's heart between the poles—for example by hooking up both your partners nipples—and as long as no one has a pacemaker. In any case, pay close attention to cardiac irregularity, the whole procedure is exciting enough in and of itself.

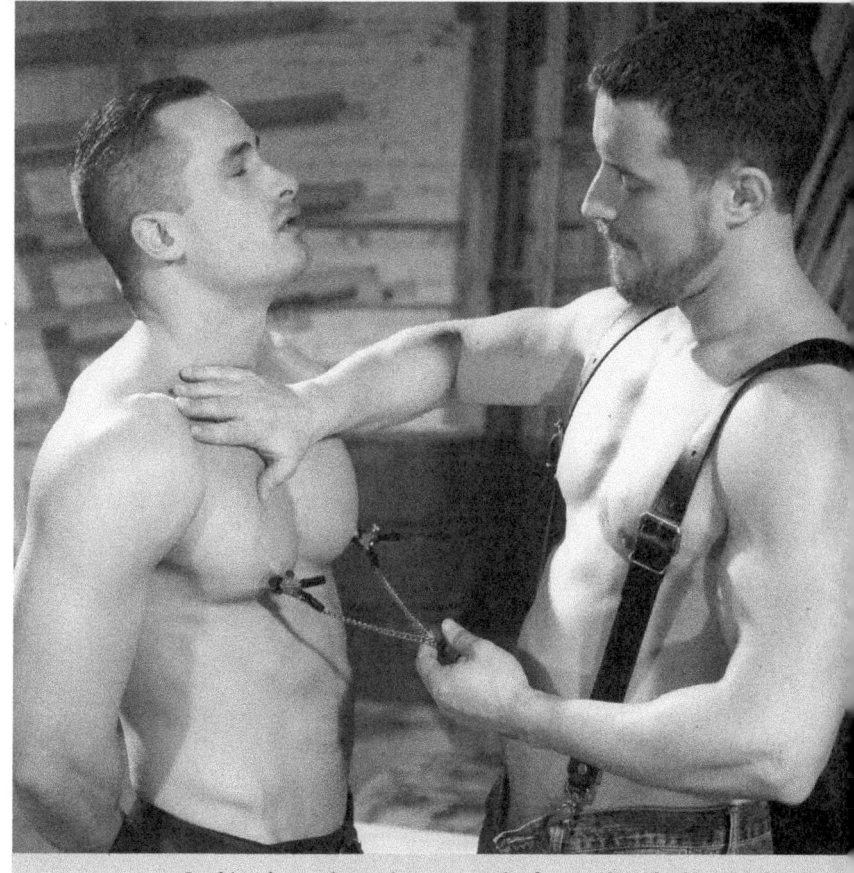

In this advanced exercise, we see the freestanding double nip-clip.

Another relatively gentle but above all inexpensive method of increasing awareness of different parts of the body and skin is provided by your good old wooden clothespin. Suction cups and nipple clamps, available from sex shops, do require a certain amount of practice. Clothespins are perfect for a first trial. They cut off the circulation in the skin. This doesn't happen right away—only after about two minutes, and it can be relatively painful, depending on how firmly the pin is attached. Before you touch the pin or the affected area, wait until the pain subsides. After removing the pin, the blood will flow back into the area, which can be just as painful as clamping. The area will remain sensitive for a while afterwards if you brush your fingers over it.

Stroking as such is still a very nice way of feeling each other, especially as painful sensations can act as an unwanted desire inhibitor. Stroking the skin hard or gently all over or in a particular place may be more appreciated. Here, too, you can defamiliarize the sensation or even intensify it. Not just with oil or other liquids on the skin, but also if you, as the "active stroker" are wearing gloves. Leather, rubber, vinyl—you can always find a model in every price range that you might like. The surprise you give your partner by grabbing his balls or rubbing his ass with a rubber glove will definitely be pain-free!

Oh, and before I forget: doesn't a cuddly blanket supplied at the end of or even during a session always guarantee cozy feelings for even the toughest guy?

▶ Interiors

Hard on the outside, soft on the inside—this applies to all men. They are all extremely soft inside: inside the mouth, inside the ass! Feeling your way inside your partner requires a special kind of trust. Penetrating the other man with your dick or your tongue, or letting him penetrate you, is considered the peak of physical closeness. It's not for nothing that the bodily openings of the mouth and anus—not to mention the cock—are on the body's axis, where both halves of the body meet, and so right in the intersection point of sensitivity.

The nerve pathways stemming from the brain cross over at the back of the neck, so that the left part of the brain governs the right half of the body and vice versa. Different abilities are attributed to the brain hemispheres: the left hemisphere is said to be the seat of rational and analytical abilities, and correspondingly, the right hemisphere is the seat of intuition and emotion. But the fact that certain factors meet in the middle and that touching, applying pressure, or penetrating them can make the greatest things happen to you, that is a given. You can feel it yourself. Letting another man into this middle–meeting another man in and at his center–that is and will always be a highlight of gay sex.

Your tongue and your dick are reliable and usually welcome body parts inside your partner. If you want to go deeper, explore his interior even further, your hand will generally be brought into play, leaving out dildos and other aids for the time being.

Does sticking the finger of your right hand (intuitive and emotional) into your partner's mouth or ass feel any different from using the left (rational and analytical)? Who cares, the main thing is that it feels good to touch the other person's center!

If penetrating and allowing oneself to be penetrated is to make anything happen in your head, the thought has to be able to get there first, so it needs to happen slowly. If you plug away immediately, the same kick can, of course, step in anyway with a short delay and perhaps even more intensity. But pain must not be allowed to destroy passion–at the most, it should curb it (see *Brotherly Pain*). So, it's all down to the right timing. Feeling your way, you will soon know how far your partner has come–in the literal sense.

If you carefully explore your partner's mouth with your hand or your fingers, you will know your boundaries soon enough, assuming he's got teeth. If he doesn't like what you're doing or if he's in pain, he can communicate this by (hopefully) gently biting down.

The anus has no teeth and so here you need to be more careful and attentive. One finger, or two –your nails should be short and filed smooth–the anus (the opening) is very sensitive to stroking or light pressure. A bit further in, and you can stimulate the prostate from inside. That happens, too, when you're fucking. This soft globe–responsible for semen production–is situated around two to three inches behind the behind the opening towards the abdominal wall.

From the outside, you can stimulate it by massaging the taint in between the balls and the anus. Some men claim that the prostate responds to stimulation like an additional sex organ. In any case handling it requires practice. If you're actively fucking, you can stimulate your own prostate by tensing the muscles in your pelvis. This can also increase your pleasure.

You want to go deeper? For this you will need gloves and a lubricant.

▷ Going Deeper

Water-based personal lubricants such as KY, Eros, or Astroglide won't damage the thin material of the disposable gloves or condoms, but Crisco and other oil-based substances (such as Vaseline) or oil will. The latter may also create tiny holes in the latex, allowing for a possible exchange of semen or blood. Water-based lubes have the disadvantage of being absorbed quickly into the skin. Regular reapplication is necessary to prevent friction. If you're planning to use a lot of it, it's worth ordering a water-based lubricant from a veterinary supply store—for example, Bovivet, which is super slippery!

Silicone-based lubricants such as Lubexxx or Swiss Navy Silicone are another alternative. The gel is based on a water-silicone mixture and lasts much longer. When using dildos or butt-plugs you should always use a condom to prevent the toy's surface from coming into contact with the gel. This can lead to a chemical reaction that cause discoloration or even partial softening in your precious toy.

Stretching the sphincter and rectum and penetrating deep into a man's interior requires great care, patience, and above all, good communication. The intense feelings resulting from deep penetration can be a challenge. How far can I go? Your partner's reactions will tell you this—that's why you need to pay attention! You need to take a cool stance towards the sort of competitive impulse and ambition that often comes into play. As long as it's enjoyable and based on mutual consent, it's a very nice way of getting close to your partner—and not just physically.

You don't necessary have to go spelunking. The surface of the skin, as described in our last chapter, also offers a wide repertoire of reactions that you can elicit, which will increase intimacy with your partner as you explore his body.

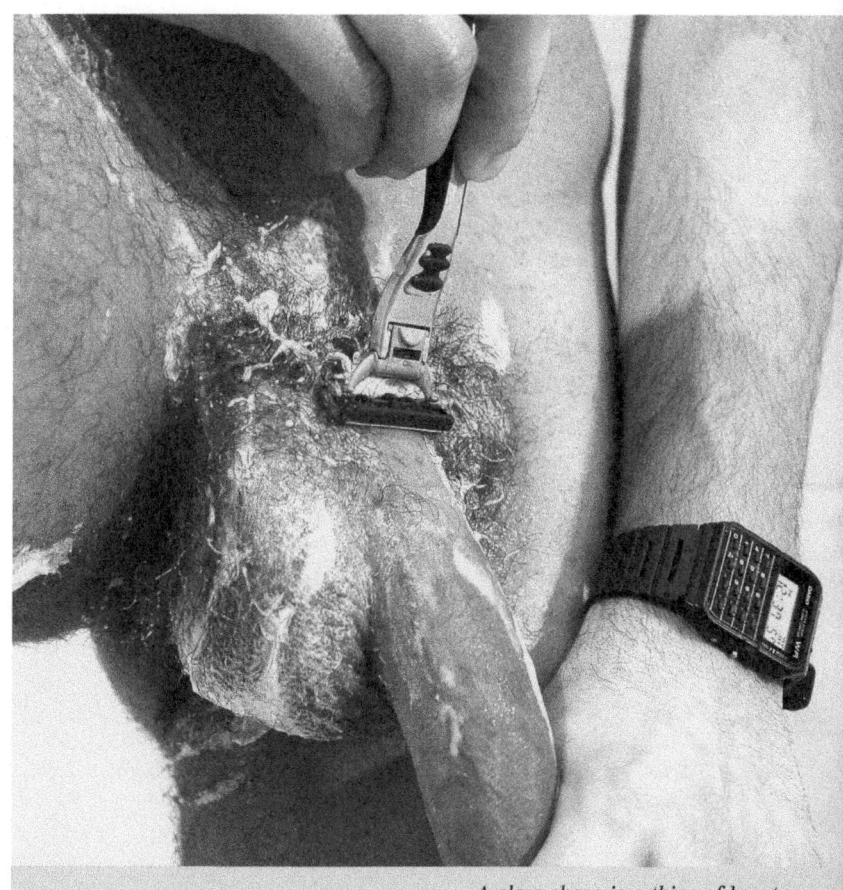

A close shave is a thing of beauty.

Slippery Games—Third Hardcore Sex Story with Bruce and Joaquin

Joaquin reclined comfortably on his back. Bruce had pulled a rope through underneath the bed and attached the ends to the leather handcuffs. Now Joaquin's arms were stretched out to the left and the right and tied fast. His feet were tied, too. A blindfold covered Joaquin's eyes so that Bruce could enjoy the sight of his naked lover at his leisure. After all the action, they both deserved a short break. Joaquin's breathing was slow and relaxed. Only his dick still twitched in an enterprising fashion and his balls appeared to move in their sac. As Bruce gazed at the two balls, he had an idea: he kissed Joaquin on the lips. "I'll be right back!" he said and left, returning shortly carrying towels, a bowl of warm water, and shaving utensils. He placed the bowl carefully next to the bed. One hand dabbled noisily in the water.

Joaquin failed to suppress a smile, but he was still unaware of what was about to happen. Now Bruce placed the towel under his partner's backside. As he began to splash water over Joaquin's dick and scrotum, Joaquin realized what Bruce was planning. His soaped-up hands slid over the exposed privates, sleeking down his skin and hair.

"That feels good," Joaquin purred.

"It will feel even better once it's all smooth!" was Bruce's reply. More splashing. Bruce washed the soap off his hands so as to get a better grip on the razor. He lifted Joaquin's slippery, semi-erect cock and placed the blade just above the first hairs that encroached on the shaft. The soft strokes left his skin smooth. Bruce took his time, cleaned off the razor with the warm water and lathered the foam around Joaquin's balls, gazing with an air of satisfaction at his partner's dick, which was slowly thickening with arousal. Then he turned to the hair on the wrinkly scrotal sac. It took several strokes of the razor before he was satisfied with the result. Apart from a patch of pubic hair, the entire area was smooth as silk. Using the water for the last time, he removed the last traces of soap. Then Bruce threw a towel into Joaquin's lap and, rubbing him hard, finished up the procedure. Now his boyfriend's dick and nut sac lay before him, spick-and-span!

The sight of Joaquin's twitching penis gave him another idea. Now that the towels were already in place ... He climbed onto the bed, stood astride the naked, bound body beneath him and leaned on the wall for support. His semi-erect cock was dangling about two feet directly above Joaquin's dick. Bruce braced his peritoneum and felt for the pressure of piss.

Yes, it was there—he felt his urethra filling up. He took a few deep breaths and then the stream splattered down from his piss hole, straight onto Joaquin's shaved junk.

Joaquin was taken by surprise by the warm shower hitting his smooth skin that his cock sprang to life right away—he was so turned on by being pissed on by another guy. The smell of the yellow swill made him even hornier, so he opened his mouth to taste the juice, to swallow it. Bruce saw his jockstrap lying on the bed, so he picked it up and held it into the stream of piss. Then he drew the wet thing over Joaquin's belly, over his chest and laid it on the other man's face. Joaquin breathed in the delicious fumes with his nose and mouth ...

▼ Take a Sniff!

Our sense of smell is the most feral of all the senses. Smells go straight to our brain stem, one of the oldest regions of the brain, without bypassing the censor. The wings of our nose follow the principle of the division of labor. They alternate every three to four hours, so that only one nostril takes in smells and air, while the other one takes a break.

The slightest traces of odor can cause a physical and emotional reaction, even if we are not consciously aware of them and without our being able to influence them. These reactions are instinctive. This varies from person to person. One man's fine perfume will disgust another man. We have a kind of olfactory memory for smells.

Odors stimulate the release of hormones that affect all bodily processes and control the entire metabolic system. We cannot prevent this from happening. Our minds are of no use to us at all here, because our sense of smell is actually seated in the limbic system, which forms part of the brain stem. This region is removed from our consciousness and thereby from our minds. It controls not only the sense of smell, but also the world of our emotions. That is why experiencing odors is a significant way of accessing areas of the subconscious.

The gag reflex that sets in whenever you smell something nasty is an example of the complexity that can be set in motion. Odors can trigger lust, but I very much doubt that you get off on the smell of incense or vanilla. In general, I would prefer to eschew herbal scents such as flowers, fruit, or herbs. They are already sufficiently well known and you can read up on them in a cookbook or elsewhere.

In perfumes, animal sources are also used, such as sex pheromones, allowing their erotic attraction to unfold over the top of a sweet or fresh scent without us being aware of them. But although I have no objections to a well-made perfume, their attractiveness has been largely dispelled. Scent is sprayed on any customer in a department store by the gallon, burying the profound impression on our senses under it. We hardly know anymore what effect a certain scent has on us and it carries no associations for us. But isn't there a forgotten world that lives on, despite this oversaturation, one that is rooted not in olfactory memory, but in a much older one, in our genetic memory?

▷ Follow Your Nose

We carry evolutionary responses to certain fragrances around with us. If you want to trigger the buried areas, the key stimuli associated with smells and reawaken them, you have to descend into the your animal depths. Forget about exquisite perfumes and discover the scent of man at his most bestial!

Tobacco, leather, and whiskey are just some of the scents associated with men. Apparently, studies have shown that cigarette smoke, for example, has an evident erotic effect. And if you don't already enjoy the scent of leather as it is, following a hot adventure involving leather, there will definitely be a lasting "scent souvenir" stored in your subconscious. This can also be achieved at will with rubber

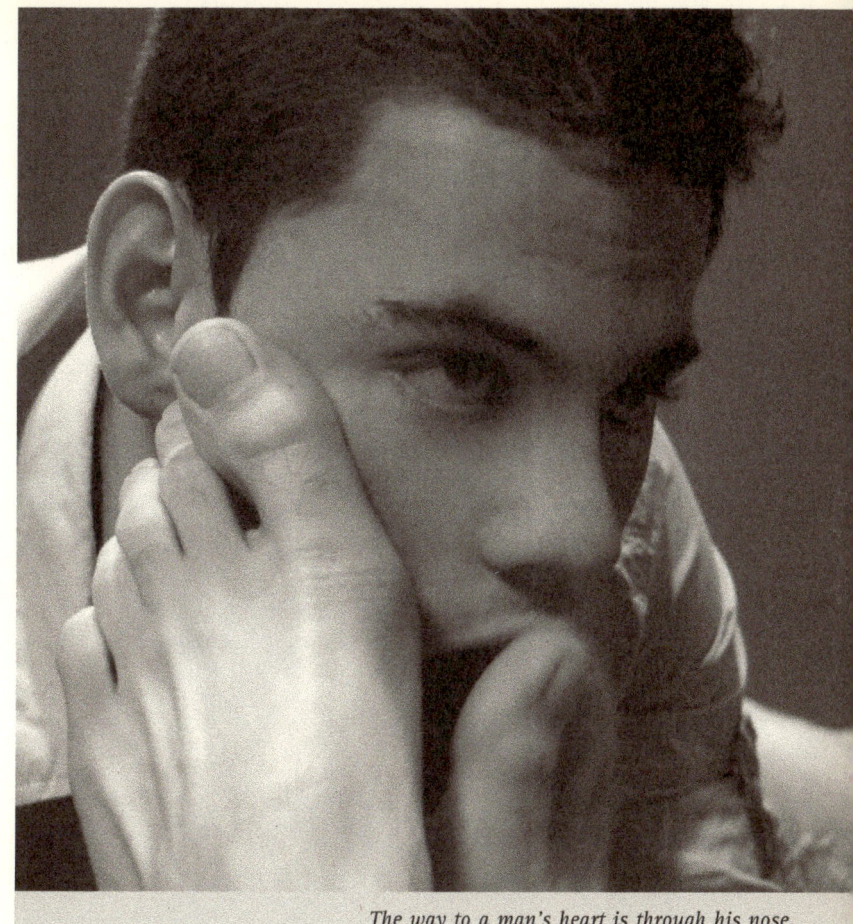

The way to a man's heart is through his nose.

or any other material. As soon as you smell this fragrance, it will stimulate your pleasure center. The degree of stimulation depends on the dose and also on any interaction with other stimuli—visual, for example, such as seeing a pair of leather boots or a rubber shirt.

In this regard, human scents function well enough without any kind of particular experience. A man is basically nothing but a large

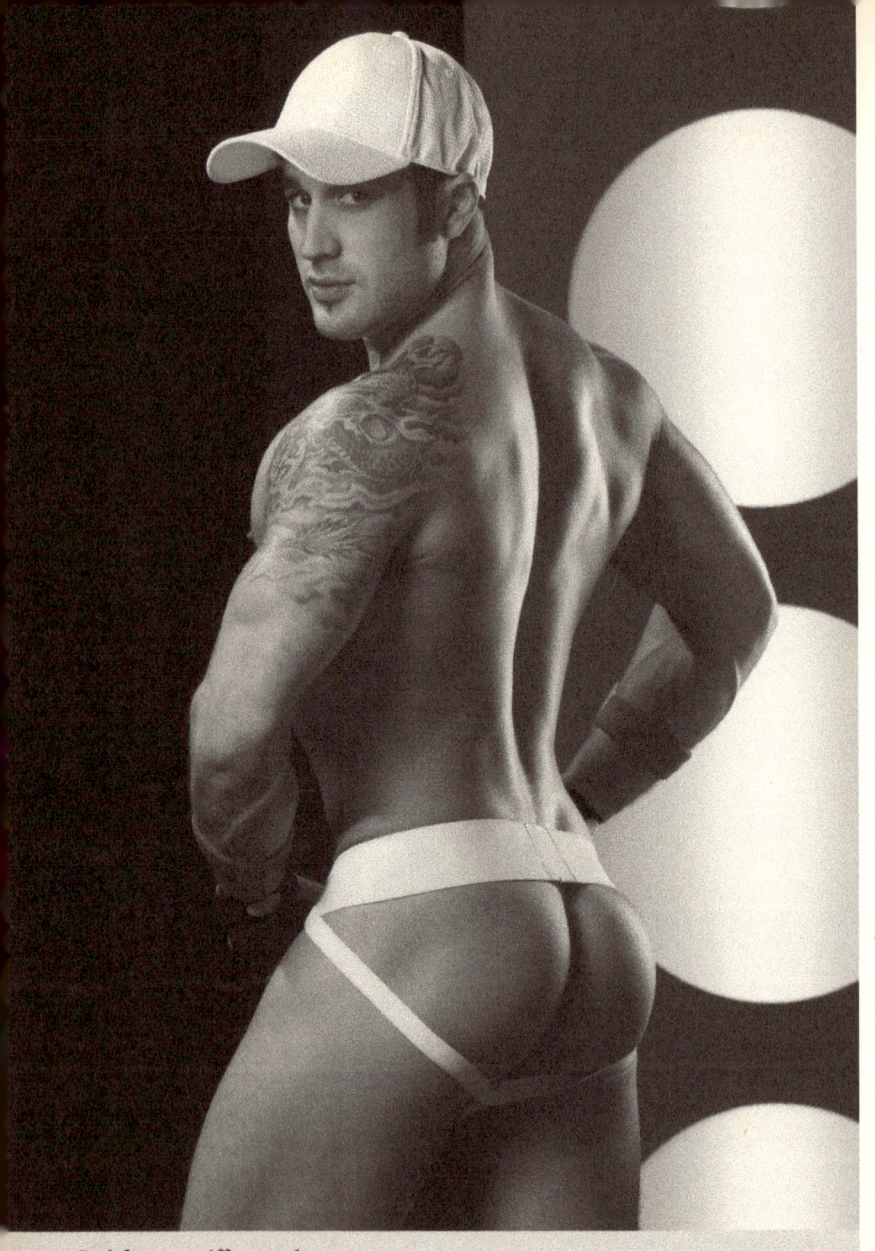

Feel free to sniff around ...

mammal, and the effect his scents have are based on ancient animal instincts. They lie in slumber outside of the realm of our consciousness. Affection, fear, trust, or mating intentions are feelings that are communicated on our interpersonal relationships by scent alone, before they have even penetrated our conscious mind through words or actions.

No matter how elegant and civilized he pretends to be, a man continually produces scents. No matter how often he washes himself or applies perfume, after a very short time his own personal scent will emerge at different points of his body. Particularly in places where there is a lot of hair and body orifices, but basically through every part of the skin.

You are well aware of your own natural smell. It's something you have to deal with and you try to cover it up and block any odor from the outside world; for in our civilized world, smelling like a human being is considered an assault. Admittedly, there are people where that is actually the case. Too many people in a confined space create too much chaos, even without a noticeable smell. So we wash, we lather ourselves up with soap, we scrub until only a minimal odor remains and there are as good as no reactions.

Can we learn to accept these suppressed sensations of smell in the private sphere and use them to increase sexual desire?

▶ Passing the Smell Test

Scents and desire go best together if you actually like your own smell. If you are disgusted by your own effluvium, you'll hardly feel like sniffing around another man, no matter how much you like or even love him. So, how do you feel about your own body odor? Do you flinch in disgust whenever you sniff at your armpit? Or can you imagine what secret messages may be hidden there? Are you embarrassed by another guy getting off on your sweat, or can you understand why he inhales great lungfuls of it?

The messages in male sweat may well be coded, but there's no need for you to think about that. Just breathe, the rest will follow. Maybe the feelings that overcome you whenever you get a noseful of that guy stem from the times when we formed packs. Perhaps fragrant proximity promotes trust. In any case, it provides a link between the transmitter and the receiver, which can significantly affect other activities. The closer you are to the source of the messenger substances, the purer the stimulus when it reaches and affects your subconscious. It Should Be Worth a Try!

It usually works best if your soap and perfume will still allow the animal part of man to permeate through. On the whole, your skin cleans itself. Sticking to washing daily and rinsing the strategically important parts of the body is usually enough to remove any dirt and to combat any really unpleasant smells. If you want your partner to be able to smell your hidden beast, you might want to leave off the deodorant, perhaps just for one day, as a surprise.

Bad breath is another matter altogether and has nothing to do with the smell of a healthy oral cavity in its normal state. The air you exhale will probably be more appreciated by your partner without interference from factors such as garlic. When you kiss, you will soon realize whether or not your scent will harmonize with that of your partner, as this is the closest two mouths will every be. This is caused by the chemical cocktail of hormones exchanged in a kiss in the sensitive tongue and cheek area which activates the production of all kinds of substances, which can in turn stimulate the immune system and general well-being, such as adrenaline and endorphins.

But what about sweat? Have you ever "bathed" in another man's sweat? Wallowed in his stink, leaving your over-civilized self behind?

Even the trauma you may have undergone merely by entering the locker room before a hated gym class can be processed with a new-found pleasure in sweat. That doesn't mean you have to smell like a barnyard. Whether it leads to sniffing your boyfriend's sweaty

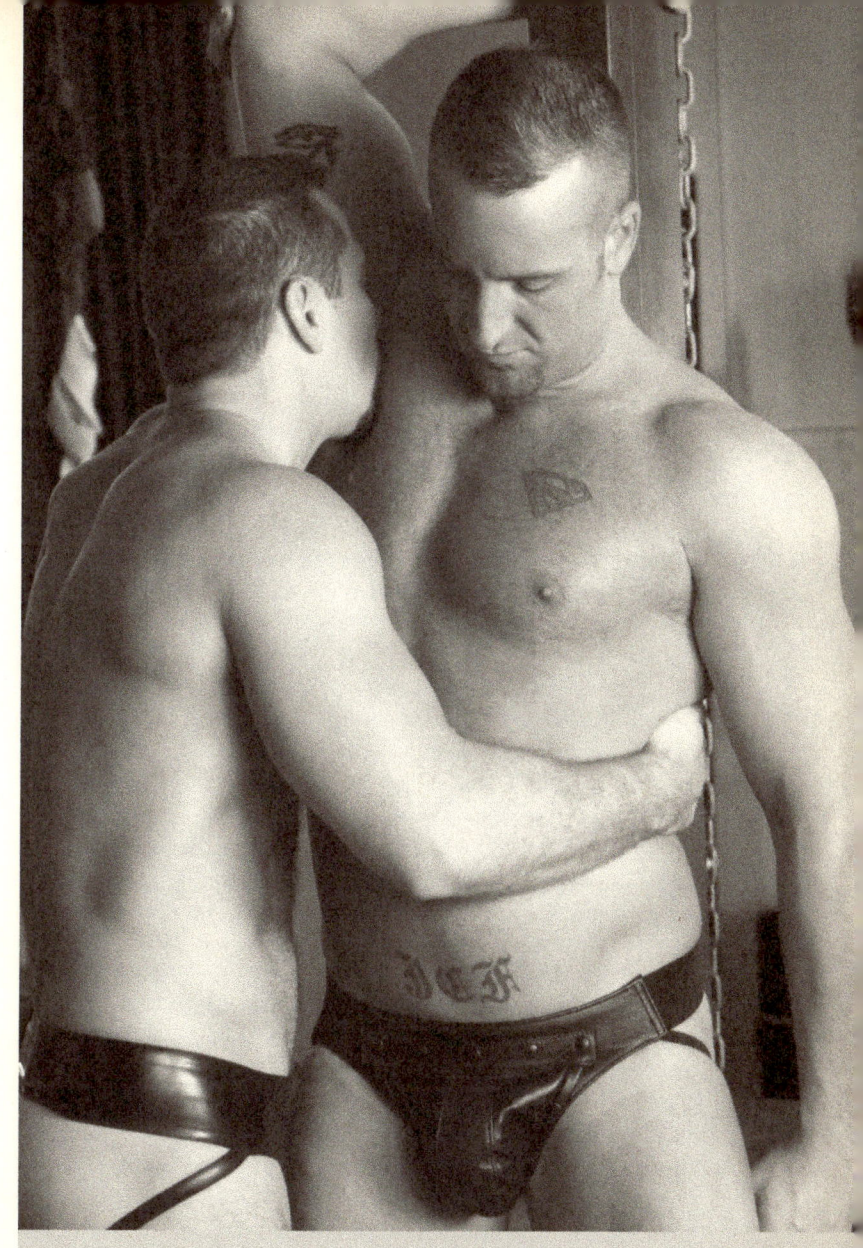

In search of encrypted messages

undershirt while you beat off or holding your own under his nose is up to you.

While you're at it: Try it out with a pair of underpants! These much lauded glands of the musk oxen produce highly effective phero-mones—similar to those of humans—and lie right in the genital area. You'll know soon enough whether or not contact with ball sweat is an eye-opener for you.

The same goes for the smell of feet or ass cracks. Not everyone's cup of tea, but an innocent enough pleasure all the same—for when we're horny and following our instincts, there's nothing more sexy than human and male.

Specialists naturally try to preserve their olfactory experiences. De-tached from an actual person, they become purely a fetish. The fact that there are no vintage series of, say, "skater sweat" available in sex shops surprises me. The aroma of a pair of worn underpants or socks can be vacuumed and/or deep frozen and brought back to life. Of course, if Mom finds a Tupperware container of socks in the deep freeze, you may have some explaining to do.

A couple of years back, I was asked to wear a pair of thin black cot-ton (!) socks for a while and then wrap them up. As the request came from a cute guy, I was happy to comply. I did my best and the next time we met, I gave him the small package. The result was disap-pointing, for even though I'd worn the things for an entire week, the fragrance was too weak for him. A more experienced friend of mine laughed at my amateurish attempts ("Ha! A week!") and then told me a joke about the new socks he had had to buy, allegedly because his old ones had broken after months of wearing.

Even without having the object before you, without even being able to smell him, the memory of certain odors and associated feelings is deeply rooted within us. If we all have an olfactory experience stored somewhere within us, can't we conjure it up again, reactivating and pleasurably reliving the memory?

▼ What Does Sex Taste Like?

I still remember the hype surrounding the movie *9½ Weeks* when it came out. The erotic food sex scenes were revolutionary. Strawberries. Sticky honey. Everything was turned into a sex aid. All of a sudden, we all wanted Mickey Rourke to squirt whipped cream into our mouths. But I'm not going to discuss food here.

Most things that smell good make you want to put them in your mouth. This is part of a survival strategy developed by us humans. Smell and taste are a well-established and experienced team. If you like the smell of something on your partner, then you will probably like the taste of it too. A perfumed armpit is not really part of your partner, its bitter soapy taste is not the revelation we are looking for here. But if the smell of his body, or part of his body turns you on, perhaps because you are aware of the intimacy that this pure sensual perception involves, then go ahead and taste it. You'll soon know whether you like it or not; your taste buds will report back to you within seconds. However, it will take a while before you know whether or not it agrees with you.

The products of a man's body are not toxic in the conventional sense of the word, but it is possible to transmit diseases. When playing with sweat and saliva, the risk is minimal. But piss and shit may result in a hepatitis infection. So, if you're into dirty sex, you need to get your vaccinations (see *Safer Sex*).

None of this sounds like a terribly inviting menu, but savoring your partner on your tongue can enhance sexual arousal. Flavor aside, saliva and sweat contain a hefty dose of hormones, a very personal mixture. When you're aroused, perspiration and salivation production are stimulated. Similar to the sense of smell, the hormone cocktail that is served to you by your partner—when kissing, for instance—sets unconscious reaction processes in motion, not the least of these being once again the production of endorphins.

How deeply you want to venture into your animal depths depends in the truest sense of the word on your personal taste. Here too, fresh sweat is a somewhat milder variation. The boundary you set between hygiene and naturalness is an individual one, but in a sexual context it can be relatively elastic.

What kinds of things does the body produce? Let's take a closer look at some of them.

Of course, boogers and earwax are also bodily products, but the penchant for these is probably limited to a very select group of fans.

Piss, on the other hand, is incorporated into a lot of sex play, not only as a pleasant shower—known as the golden shower—but it also finds its way into the gaping beaks of many a thirsty goldfinch, outside of the frequently recommended but controversial urotherapy. Piss con-

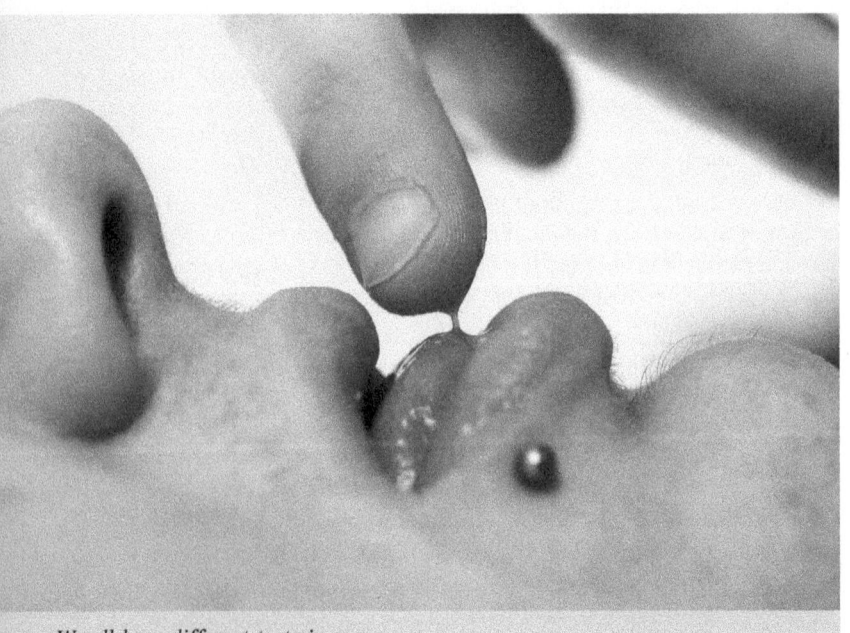

We all have different taste in men.

sists of ninety-five percent water. Apart from salts, urea, uric acid, and other metabolic waste products, it also contains small amounts of sugar, as well as a whole lot of hormones and fragrances that can have strong effects. In a healthy human being, the urine stored in the bladder is sterile. Only when passing through the lower portion of the urethra can it come into contact with germs. It is therefore advisable not to swallow the first stream right away. The comparison with broth is surprisingly apt, not only because of the salts it contains, but also because its pH-values are in the acidic region. After the first stream, the taste of piss is more neutral, depending on what drinks or food have been consumed. Why asparagus has such a devastating effect on the taste and smell of piss is a question I am happy to leave up to those of you who are really thirsty for knowledge.

Feces consists, among other things, of the indigestible components of your diet, other residues such as fats and starch, as well as water. It gets its color from bile pigments and its smell from the byproducts formed when proteins are digested, for example hydrogen sulfide. Fungi and bacteria are the reason for a certain level of risk to your health.

Smegma, also known as dick cheese, is a whitish-to-pale yellow substance that is produced by the sebaceous glands between the foreskin and the glans. Other components of this greasy paste are, apart from gland secretions, urine and sperm residue as well as loads of bacteria. It's a kind of natural ointment that keeps the sensitive areas of the genitals lubricated, but in these hygienic times it is no longer that popular, especially because of the unpleasant smell.

Apart from water, semen contains a load of salts, proteins (the sperm itself) and hormones, including testosterone, pheromones, and endorphins. Whether ingesting it actually acts as an antidepressant, as American studies claim, is definitely not due to the tiny amount of gold, which also is found in semen. The mushroomy smell comes from spermine, a polyamide that strengthens the sperm's DNA. Just as with piss, medications such as antibiotics have a strong influence on the odor and taste of semen.

The alkaline taste of so-called pre-cum, produced by the bulboure-thral glands before ejaculation and passed through the urethra to clean it, is also a purely male affair, and therefore sensational.

A man's molecular cuisine is pretty inventive and constantly in motion. In any case, your table is ready, sir! Shouldn't we tear off the tablecloth and the dishes of perfume and soap and enjoy some really good sex on its own?

Lickety Split—Third Softcore Sex Story with Brad and Corey

Home at last! The trip home had stretched out, interrupted by numerous making-out sessions in entryways and front yards. Even in the bar, Corey had noticed the pungent male smell that Brad exuded, and it was really turning him on. He was glad he had persuaded Brad not to apply deodorant before they hit the bar. The scent of fresh sweat acted on Corey like an aphrodisiac—especially today, though he had no idea why.

When they came in through the door, Corey slipped under his boyfriend's armpit once more and sniffed into the damp fabric of his T-shirt. One hand between Brad's legs confirmed that he was just as aroused.

Indeed, Brad was turned on by his boyfriend unrestrained intoxication from his sweat. He raised his other arm and pushed the other guy's head into his armpit, giving him the full dosage. The heady scent rose into his own nostrils. Not bad at all! He grinned. It had been a good idea to keep the soapy stick out of his pits, positively liberating! Without Corey knowing it, Brad hadn't been using the thing for a while now. He had realized that a daily shower and freshly laundered clothes were perfectly sufficient. Apart from that, he now preferred his own smell, even during the day, and he loved Corey's natural body odor.

As soon as they were inside, he took off Corey's T-shirt, pushed him up against the wall, pulled both naked arms up by the wrists and stuck his tongue in his lover's hairy pits, first one, then the other. It tasted delicious! Corey disentangled himself and tore off Brad's shirt. Then his tongue began its search for the salty place under his boyfriend's arms, slithered over the trimmed hairs and felt the scent hit his nose and taste buds. Mmmm! They combined their fluids in a passionate kiss and tasted each other.

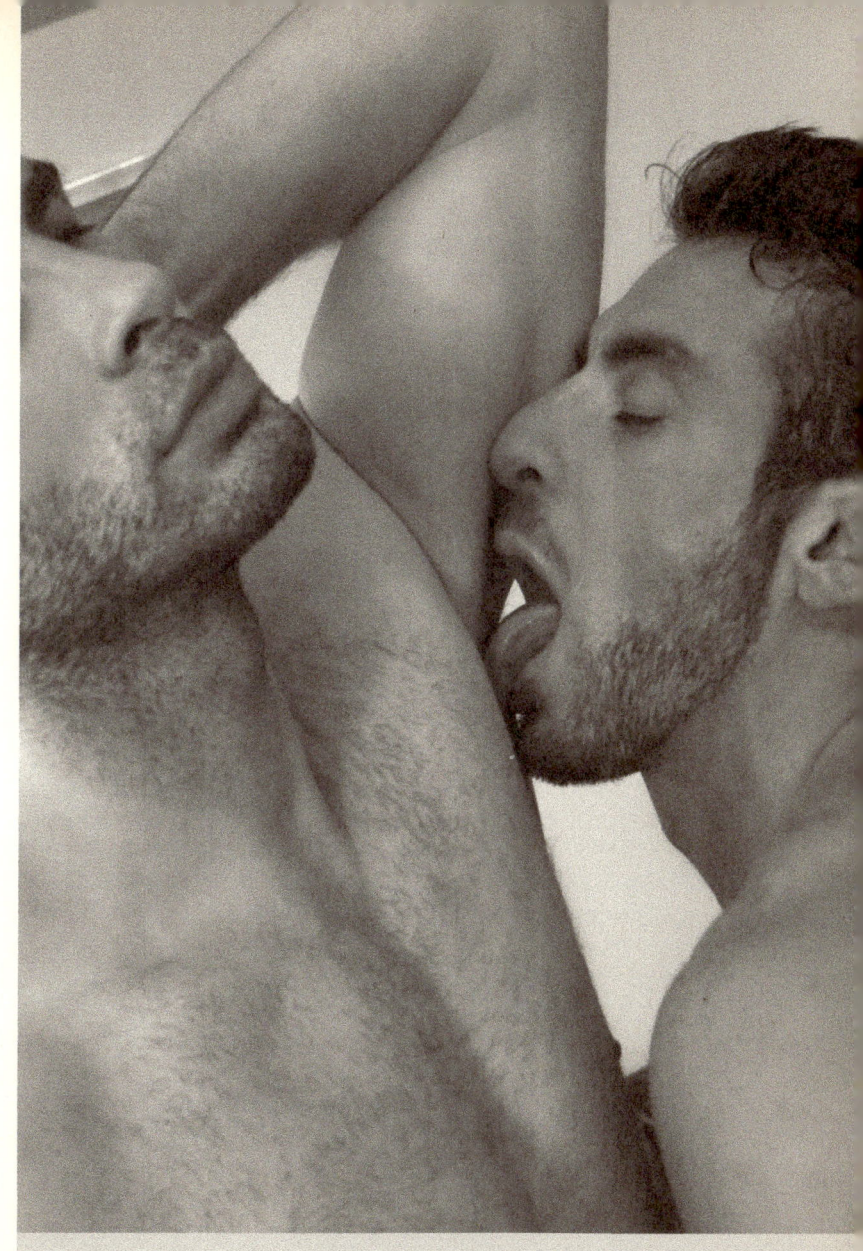

Scent of a man: the all-natural high

As Corey went down on his knees in front of Brad, he could barely wait to finally reach the bulge in his pants. He unbuttoned his jeans and sniffed noisily at the underpants that gleamed white through the fly. Only after he had licked wetly over the place where the fabric covered his balls a few times could he smell the scent of Brad's nut sac over the light tang of the laundry detergent. Or maybe he was imagining it. Corey could also smell a whiff of ammonia—the residue of a couple of drops of piss that had gone into his pants. He would have liked to ask his boyfriend to wear the same underpants for a few days so that they could really take in his smell, but he didn't have the guts.

At the moment, he was overcome by anticipation for Brad's dick that was outlined, firm and swollen, under the cotton fabric. Once he had pulled Brad's sturdy pecker out from inside his underpants, he wanted to make a grab for it right away and stuff it in his mouth. But he restrained himself, deciding to take it slow and enjoy the anticipation. He took pleasure in the sight of the hard muscular shaft jutting out of his pants. The shaft, with its velvety skin stretched over the erect tissue, the part underneath where the glans tugged at the frenulum. The entire thing seemed to radiate heat, as if it had its own aura! Corey sucked in a lungful of air. It was pregnant with the pungent smell of dick.

Corey looked up at Brad, meeting his gaze while he sniffed downwards from the tip to the balls, only occasionally touching the skin with the tip of his tongue, so as to take in every part of his scent with every nerve. Brad bathed in his horny gaze, transported by the arousing connection between him and his lover that lay in the air. He sent down a thread of spit and it landed on the smooth glans. Corey stuck out his tongue to catch the viscous drop. It felt like licking semen off of Brad's dick. He pushed his head between Brad's legs, under his balls, and rubbed his stubbly head on his boyfriend's junk. Brad grinned. It tickled! He spread his legs to give Corey's head better access. Corey tore down his pants off his ass and worked his way—following his nose—into the crack. He breathed stertorously as the first dank whiff hit him. Going for another man's ass gave him a tremendous kick. The shamelessness, the breach of a taboo, maybe even the animal side of it—didn't dogs sniff around each other's backsides all the time?—he wasn't interested in clearing that up. All he knew was how hot it was to explore this intimate zone with his nose, with his tongue. He had hardly run his tongue once through the crack, before Brad turned around.

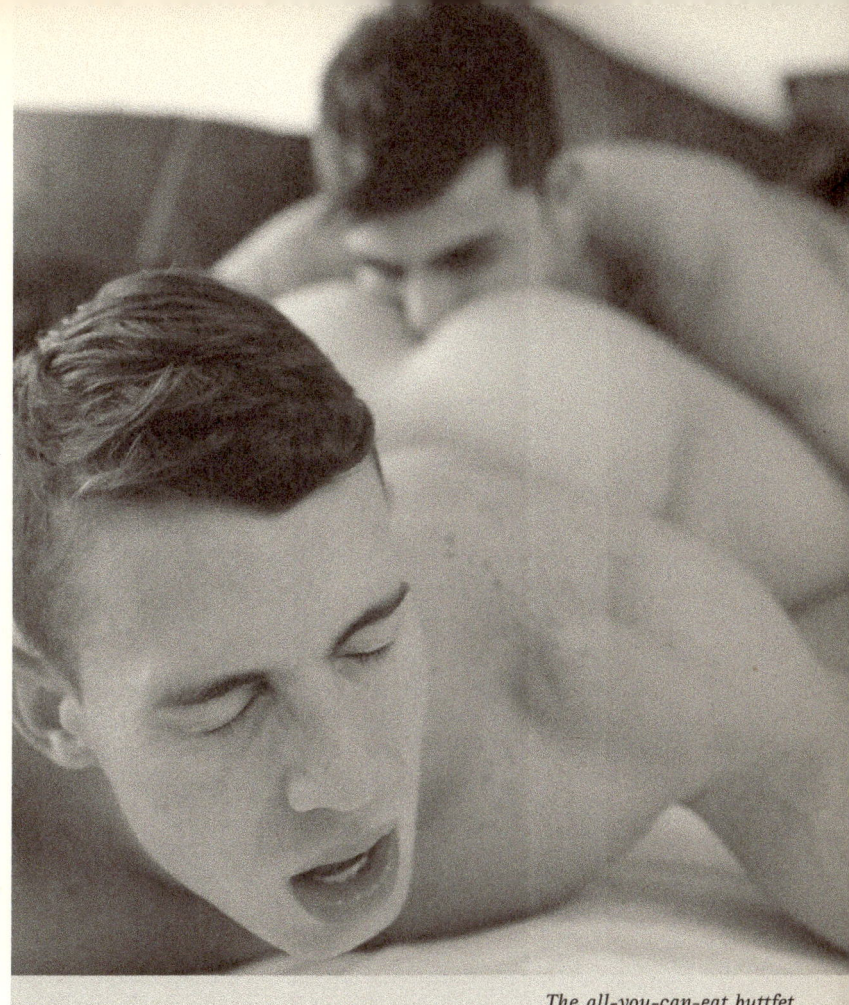

The all-you-can-eat buttfet

Before Corey even had time to register disappointment, Brad directed his attention towards the pre-cum that had formed on the tip of his cock. With circling motions of his tongue, Corey lapped up the salty drop and led Brad feed him more of it. Then Brad turned his strapping ass back to him. Corey didn't have to be asked twice. This time he slapped one of the cheeks with his right hand, then again. It was louder than he'd expected.

▼ Can You Hear Who's Coming?

Playing with your sense of hearing is difficult during sex. Apart from background music, it is rarely triggered. If it's obstructed or turned off completely—for instance with earplugs—this results in a strange feeling because your sense of hearing is in close proximity to your sense of balance. If we can hear, then what we hear can still stimulate or inhibit desire.

While talking to Roland, a friend from Cologne, about sex yet again, he told me "I need to hear the guy cum!" In bed, he meant. Soon after, he came to visit me in Munich and stayed at my place. I fell asleep to the screams of the guy he'd brought home from the bar and woke up the next morning to more of the same. Roland was apparently nailing his sex partner so hard, the other guy couldn't help but scream out his pleasure with increasing volume and in a constant staccato. Every time I thought it was over, it started up again!

I could kind of get why Roland always had trouble with the neighbors back in Cologne. My own neighbors were nice enough the next morning and gave me a friendly hello at the mailbox, as if they had not spent the night with sound effects straight from the delivery ward.

While all the screaming would have been too much for me personally, I still know what Roland meant.

If we're not actually doing it in the changing room of a department store, there is no reason to act like we're in a silent movie. Along with those guys who never move during sex, the mute ones are another example of guys that are no fun to have sex with, because sex isn't a silent affair. Sex involves noise. The level of noise you want during sex is up to you. But if you can't hear a thing? Then it sounds as if there's nobody there. It's better to communicate how turned on you are to your partner non-verbally, and get him carried away too! Moan, purr, and slobber! Particularly if a certain position or situation is extremely hot, a few well-placed sounds can make that clear.

The same goes, of course, if there's anything you don't like. You don't have to make an exaggerated amount of noise, but suppressing a smack or a slurp during whatever you're doing will dampen your passion more than stimulating it. The volume will adapt to the natural flow of action. It can also be your sole means of communication. The more unrestrained the sex, the more unrestrained the level of noise can be. Now you know!

The interplay of sound and lust during sex only gets really interesting if you can't see anything. If you're blindfolded, every sound gets its own personal interpretation and is associated with images in your head. If they aren't directly connected to what's happening with your body, they create a puzzle and increase the suspense. This is especially rich in variety if you're using different materials or toys while you're having sex. Their introduction into play can be announced by sounds, for example the click of a pair of handcuffs. But the sounds you make in everyday actions or footsteps can also suddenly start off a movie inside your head. A beer bottle being opened. For him? For you? Are you going to be given a drink? From the bottle? From his mouth? As the active partner, you can pick up on the expectations that arise.

The Listening Game—Fourth Hardcore Sex Story with Bruce and Joaquin

Joaquin strained to interpret the rattling noise he had just heard. He lay in the sling. Bruce had covered his eyes with a soft leather blindfold. Bruce laughed and bent down, as Joaquin could tell from the creaking of his leather pants. Something metallic had fallen onto the wooden floor. A cock ring? No, it sounded lighter than that. The nipple clamps? He could hear Bruce's footsteps approaching in their heavy boots, and felt him step in between his legs that were held apart by the sling. Fingers touched his mouth and nose. Joaquin stuck out his tongue and tried to lick them. Now something was held under his nose. It smelled of beer. When the thing touched his lips, he flinched. It had sharp edges! "Stick out your tongue!" came the command from Bruce.

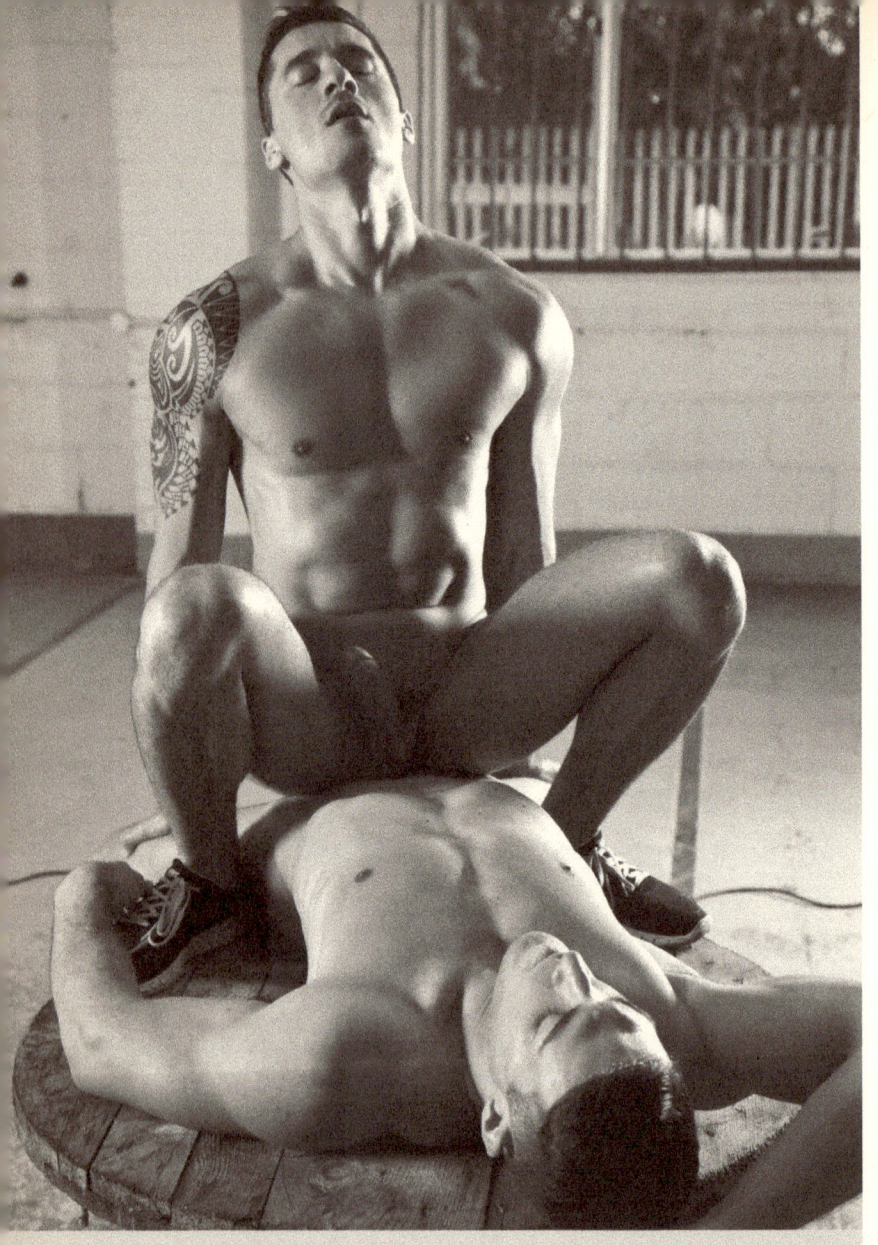

New position: "How's this for easy access?"

Carefully Joaquin pushed the tip of his tongue through his barely parted lips, explored the object and soon realized that it was just a bottle cap. Why should he lick a bottle cap? But then the object moved gently down his chin, scraping slightly down his neck and ending up on his right nipple. Just a little more pressure and Joaquin could distinctly feel the crown of thorns on his skin. Bruce moved the pressure around in circles, increased it, pushing the nipple flat while the spikes bit into the skin. Joaquin moaned and involuntarily pushed his pelvis towards the man standing between his legs. The pressure decreased.

Like a cogwheel, Bruce rolled the bottle across his chest to the other side. He did the same thing to the left nipple. Joaquin groaned again. Even while attempting to concentrate on what he was feeling at the moment, he still asked himself—somewhat fearfully—what Bruce was planning to do with it next.

But then, after rolling it over his belly, Bruce laid the bottle cap down over his navel. With broad strokes his tongue lapped at the irritated nipples and the warm wetness felt good. Now he could feel Bruce's dick at his anus. It was slippery enough, the thick prong easily found its way inside his boyfriend. Again, Joaquin moaned, drawn-out, luxurious moans. He could feel the spit drying on his chest, leaving only a slight burning sensation in his nipples. The feeling in his ass was more important now!

▼ Switching Gears

Changing over from one part of the body to the next will create an awareness for your body, just as switching over from one sense to the next will make you aware of your senses. Both are important for good sex, whether you intend to focus on one thing in particular, or prefer a potpourri—in the long run, it depends on the length of time you and your partner choose for what you do together. It takes time for your feelings to adjust to the change, and you need to give yourself that time. Turning stimuli on and off causes a bodily reaction that doesn't have to have any sort of profound reason. Your subconscious will take care of it on its own. You can only let it happen if stimulation is followed by relaxation.

Total sensory deprivation, the suppression of all the senses, such as being forced to sit, stand or lie down tied up, gagged, blindfolded and wearing earplugs is the province of experienced S&S practitioners. It is also used as a torture and interrogation method and can cause hallucinations and cognitive disorders. The insertive partner needs to know a lot about the other man's physical and emotional constitution. A firm basis of trust between both partners is necessary if the closed-off partner's total focus on his inner being is to lead to an expansion of consciousness.

As a rule, sex will consist of other things than dumping a guy in a corner like a wrapped up package. It will not only involve the interplay of the senses we have just described—sex between the two of you will also be determined by other factors. The speed with which you kickstart your arousal curve, for example, before you let it die down and start it up again, or reach a climax, or the mood you create for the action you have planned. The longer you are together sexually, the more arousing a change can be, from fast to slow, light to dark, soft to hard. Isn't it the transition from one extreme to the next that raises the experience into the realm of consciousness, turning it into a lasting and incredibly hot memory?

___ A Recipe for Good Sex (Ingredients)

▼ Movement and Standstill

People react differently to the same stimulus, depending on the situation, but all the same, there are a couple of universally applicable points. Familiar sensations have their own charm. They are recognizable and can have a calming and relaxing effect. Unfamiliar sensations, on the other hand, will engage your attention and can have a stimulating effect. The alternating use of both types of sensation will have an effect on the sexual suspense curve. If everything moves at the same pace, it rarely leads to a revelation.

Taking a rest, breaking up the rhythm, identifying and enjoying climaxes, avoiding over-stimulation—all of this takes practice. But practicing is fun, after all! It's all about finding out what's best for you or the other person.

When you're fucking, regular thrusts can feel pleasant or annoying. Are you stressed and having to put out fires everywhere in your job? After about the twentieth thrust in the ass at the same rhythm, pressure, and angle, you'll have grasped the pattern and you can relax and wait for the next push, or thrust yourself; the struggle is over. Or maybe the monotonous pounding is getting on your nerves, not distracting you enough from your problems and shifting your focus on other things.

Are you a bundle of nerves, charging about restlessly all the time? Let yourself be pushed into the mattress with a deep thrust until you stop thrashing and your center is completely immobilized and see how good that feels! On the other hand, if you need to let off steam, then you'll be needing more action than that.

Alternating between movement and standstill is a good way of experimenting with passion. Good sex involves a certain balance between action and tranquility, perfectly suited to the moment.

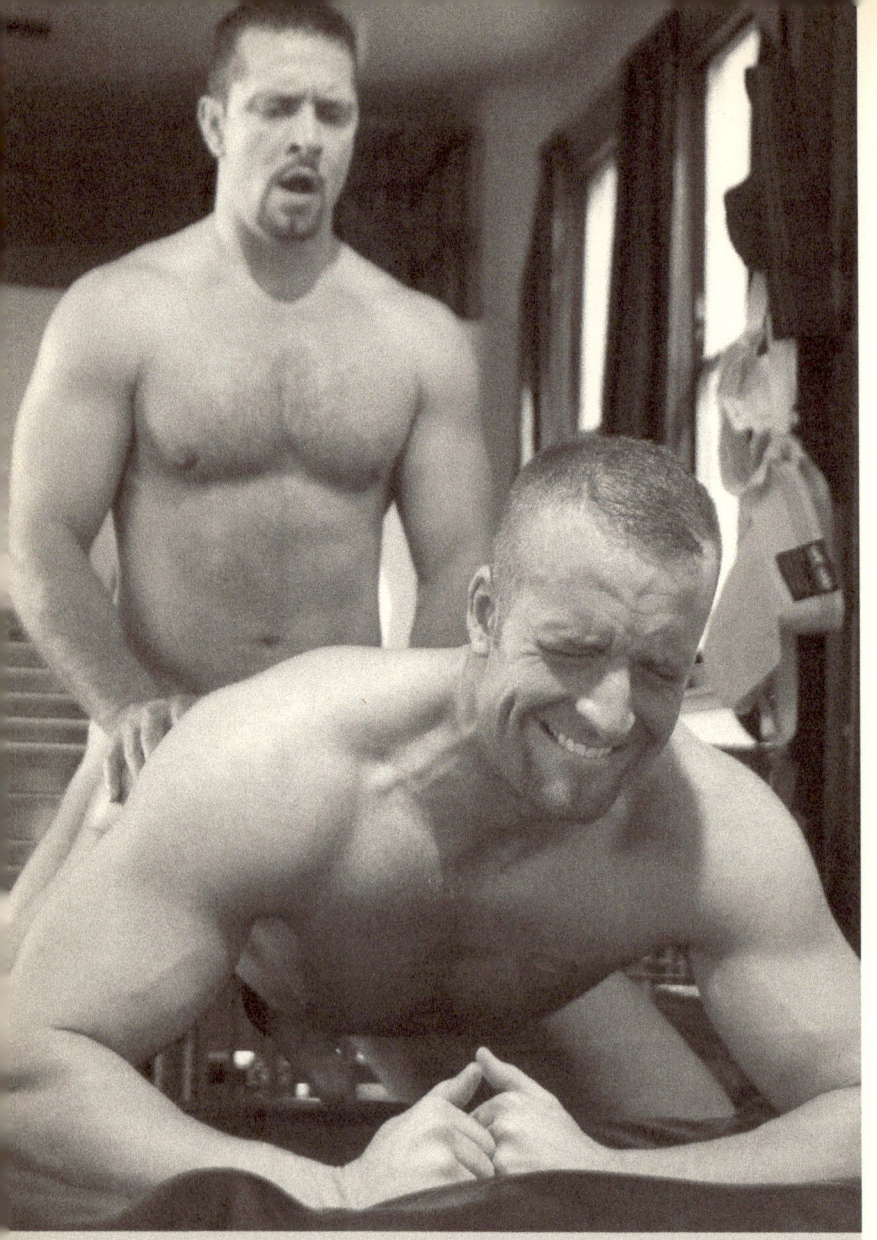

With slow strokes he rams his fat cock into the tight hole.

Nailing it—Fourth Softcore Sex Story with Brad and Corey

Brad kneeled behind Corey on the bed. With slow strokes, he rammed his thick cock into the tight hole. In, out, in, out, he was in no hurry. When Corey pushed his pelvis towards him in excitement, wanting more sensation, getting more and more worked up, Brad moved up and lay down on top of him with all his weight, pressing him down flat on the mattress, soothing him, then took his arms and stretched them out to either side, stroked his upper arms, forearms, and hands. With his thighs, he pushed Corey's legs together, felt for his feet with his own and touched them. They lay on top of each other as if crucified. Brad was enjoying the friction of Corey's tight ass on his cock while Corey could feel the pressure deep inside him. Gently, very gently, Brad pressed his pelvis further into the backside underneath him, pushing his dick just a few millimeters further into the heat of Corey's body. It took all of Corey's strength to brace himself against the pressure, against the hard peg impaling him, but he tried to all the same. Trembling with arousal and exertion, he waggled his ass around on the bed, so as to feel the connection with Brad more intensely. The heat inside him increased more and more until it felt like he was smoldering in the place where his ass muscles were closed tight around the shaft. The body lying on top of him didn't yield—it nailed him deeper and deeper into the mattress and seemed to get heavier and heavier. Corey couldn't move a thing—neither his arms, nor his legs, back, ass or belly—everything was pinned down by the bodyweight of the man whose thick cock was stuck deep inside his ass. Corey surrendered.

After a while, his gasps slowed down, his breathing became deeper and more regular until he felt himself breathing in the same rhythm as Brad with his weight on his body. As they both rocked up and down, gently, almost imperceptibly, he felt his own tension ease. His muscles relaxed, a languorous feeling took hold of him, beginning with the fire in the middle of his body, inside his ass. His excitement abated, even the pressure in his dick subsided and he felt the pleasant rush of blood in his veins. His pulse slowed and it felt as if his beating heart was expanding. It was like being high! Brad listened for Corey's breathing and grinned when he heard him purring like a kitten. He stroked the slack limbs—no longer needing the other man's weight, having accepted their own heaviness—and began to use a circling motion to increase the sensation within Corey's ass, until he finally pulled out, drew back, and shoved his dick back in. Corey no longer tried to reach for it greedily, he was content to lie there, hold out his box, and let himself be fucked hard. His contented expression and languorous groans spoke volumes. That wasn't so hard, was it?

▷ Men and Movement

Men allegedly have a greater urge to move than do women , at least that's what they say. See the often-cited comparison between women as gatherers and men as hunters. The gatherer crawls about, crouching, concentrating on a particular goal, berries for example, while the hunter seeks out the open spaces, ranging across the world, his attention directed everywhere, for instance towards the next mammoth. Pretty strenuous!

Then there are the male archetypes of air and fire. Air corresponds to noise. Fire is fast and frenzied. Intensity, ecstasy, dance, and travail are the male, fiery aspects of dynamism. Their effects extend to "burning up" anxiety, dissolving inhibitions and obstructions. Everyone has experienced the rush of speed and the feeling of liberation it evokes.

Perhaps it is the male hormone testosterone that is responsible for men charging about through time and space. Male adolescents have approximately five times more of this hormone in their bodies than females, adult men have on average several times as much as women. Testosterone is allegedly responsible not only for increasing sexual desire, but also for burning fat and building up muscle mass. With the right amount of this in his blood, a guy has no choice but to race about so as to burn up fatty tissues and build up muscle mass. The hormone needs an outlet. So you go skating or jogging, work out at the gym, ride your motorcycle into the setting sun, dance till you're tired, or just beat off like a maniac. As long as you keep the fires stoked and the engines running at full blast.

And yet, every man yearns for peace and quiet. Of course, rest is not seen as a bad thing, but it does mean inactivity and is associated with feelings of guilt, when every man is expected to be as active as possible and to keep his life firmly in hand. Even relaxation exercises or yoga do require activity. They have to be learned and then practiced. You yourself are responsible for doing this, guilt and frustration are your constant companions. Can't someone come over and just switch off the engine?

▷ Men at Rest

Aside from masochists who draw pleasure from being tied up and immobilized and then painfully struggle against it, there are men who are able to just surrender and enjoy an enforced physical passiveness. It may even give them a feeling of freedom, the ability to come to rest and concentrate on themselves. The bonds of liberty, so to speak—whether or not they can be traced back to our oft-cited feeling of well-being within the womb, like floating in a closed tank of salt water. The ultimate goal is "cocooning," the feeling of absolute security, as if wrapped up in a cocoon. In any case, the conscious and total restriction of your ability to move is a gift not to be found on every man's wish list, but everyone should ask himself once in a while, whether it might not do him some good.

Rope play, bondage, and mummification, then. You don't have to jump straight into full-body bondage. Try simply putting someone's hands out of action by tying them with fabric ties or leather cuffs or fixing them somewhere, and you're good to go. In contrast to just holding on to someone's hands, which generally happens only briefly and can be stopped quickly and easily, tying someone up requires one partner to surrender himself to the other guy. Before you tie up your partner, or let him tie you up, it can be helpful to take what's next on the program into account. If you're tied up sitting on a chair, your ass won't be part of the action. Tied standing up against the wall, your partner's mouth will be out of reach unless there's a way for you to get up to the same level, by climbing on a sturdy chair, for instance.

The breadth of materials at your disposal offers a number of visual and tactile variations. Professional gear such as straitjackets or body bags is not really suitable for anyone with only a passing interest, especially once you consider the price. Soft nylon ropes, chains, and hooks are readily available and can make a good starter kit. Very long ropes are more difficult to work with than shorter ones. Robust clingfoil or duct tape, the silver, cotton-backed tape they use in film productions, can also be used to restrain limbs or attach them to something. This can extend to completely wrapping someone up, mummifying them to the point that hardly any sexual interaction is possible. The mental kick that can be achieved by this is restricted to the patient and experienced, as the procedure takes a long time and everything has to fit exactly right, so as not to obstruct circulation and breathing.

If it didn't have such esoteric connotations, I could imagine drumming playing a part here in slowing down the pulse rate. According to some theories of music, this would involve rhythms that get men keyed up, such as techno or a ternary meter, like you'd hear in a waltz. I'm not so sure about techno, though. After all, this musical style is widely used in all the important events in the gay fetish scene as "fucking music." But the mere thought of being immobilized, shoved into a sack and forced to listen to André Rieu at peak volume makes me break out into a sweat. Now the term "demon fiddler" makes perfect sense to me! That must be what hell is like! Perhaps it would be preferable to have no music, no sounds at all, and be able to fully concentrate on one's inner being.

Certain agreements should be made in advance, but I would advise against embarking on these kinds of games without a halfway experienced partner. It goes without saying that a great deal of trust is necessary for the receptive partner to experience his total immobilization as a voyage into the light. The bound person will be able to completely surrender up his mobility only if his immobilization is supervised— that is to say with a constantly present and attentive partner. This can result in an actual high, and once you've seen the happy face of a man following the procedure, that's all the incentive you'll ever need.

Unless he would rather go wild, burn up testosterone, blow, fuck, and jerk off! Can a man even ejaculate with all this rope and bondage play going on?

Accessing Your Man

For the person doing the tying-up, the attraction lies in your partner's surrender. Submitting to the bondage, the power imbalance that this creates, the visualization through the materials you have chosen, looking forward to what you can "simply" go ahead and do with the other person, even the aesthetic aspect of the sight of a bound man, all of this can be pleasurable. Considering the amount of work involved, the idea of being dominant has to be seen in perspective, because you do have to work hard at it to get the right results. That is why it is advisable to focus on the journey rather than the destination. The body's slow and gradually induced surrender into passiveness can be interrupted at any time by sexual or tender acts. The results can vary too, according to need.

If certain parts of the body are accessible without the bound partner being able to defend himself, then you can add erotic domination into the mix. After all, the point of the entire exercise is to let you use his body without hindrance. His mouth, nipples, dick, balls, and ass are especially fun to play with, but that depends on your preferences. If your tied-up partner is also blindfolded, you can take your time and turn your attention to his erogenous zones, even in a brightly lit setting, without the pressure of looking good yourself.

Depending on how you choreograph the action, you can gradually increase his immobility until he is completely restrained, or let alternating intervals of rest and action determine your rhythm. Giving the bound partner the time he needs to adapt to his conditions and relax, letting him embark on a journey into his innermost self, is

Men in Bags—An Interview with Olaf

Olaf, aged thirty-three, is a good-looking man with a shaved head and a body bursting with strength. He's into mummification. I asked him what he liked about being wrapped up in a helpless bundle and placed at the mercy of another man.

▸ **What's the appeal of bondage and mummification?**
Olaf: Giving up all responsibility. All day long, my head is full of all the things I have to or want to do. If I'm not forced to switch off, I just can't relax.

▸ **So, you need it from time to time?**
Definitely! There's a certain time period it has to happen in for me to feel myself. About every couple of weeks.

▸ **With partners you know well?**
Well, that's kind of debatable. Under some circumstances it's enough for me to briefly get to know the other person before we get down to business. You develop a pretty good feeling for whether or not it might work out.

▸ **Even with complete strangers?**
That may be a really hot fantasy, but carrying it out would definitely not end well.

▸ **Is the main point of your act the bondage and wrapping you up?**
Basically it's about being made helpless—especially if I'm physically stronger than my partner. As long as I know that I can defend myself, there are some things I won't allow to be done to me.

▸ **For example?**
If I'm to get a beating, then it has to made clear beforehand that I will be prevented from hitting back. That's the only way it makes sense to me.

▸ **So, you're not that submissive?**
(Laughs) Nah, not really. That's exactly the point!

▶ **What are the requirements for the session to work at all?**
Definitely a mutual liking. And, of course, there has to be a spark, too. I
also need to feel that I am respected as a person. After all, I am in total
surrender.

▶ **How does a typical session start out?**
Well, first I need time to warm up. I can't get in to my car straight after
work and then right into the bag. I also need to know that there's no time
pressure. In theory, my surrender has to be able to go on for a long time.
The idea is for the active partner to decide when I can be my own master
again, and that's when he wants me to, and not as determined by external
circumstances. If I know that I have yet another social obligation in two
hours, or similar, I can't let myself go.

▶ **What happens during your warm-up time?**
My favorite time for this is the weekend, where we have the time to talk a
bit about everything that's about to happen. A bit of a cuddle beforehand
isn't bad, either.

▶ **Do you prefer certain materials?**
They all have their own appeal. The main thing for me is that I end up totally immobilized. It's easiest if I am wrapped up in clingfoil, for example,
on a bench.

▶ **So you're not suspended in space?**
That would give me too much freedom of movement. I prefer being fas-
tened to something.

▶ **What about your eyes and mouth?**
I'm am usually blindfolded. It's also important to me to have a proper gag, a
piece of fabric stuck in my mouth and then taped up so that I can't scream
or make any intelligible sounds.

▶ **What happens when you lie there all wrapped up?**
I shut down completely. I'm totally relaxed because I know that there is absolutely nothing I can do at the moment.

▶ **What do you do if something starts to hurt after all the wrapping up?**
You have to pay attention to that from the very beginning. For example, if my shoulder starts to hurt after a while, then I can't concentrate on the pain being inflicted on me deliberately in another place.

▶ **So, there is some physical action?**
Well yes, but it depends on my partner's mood. Sometimes nothing happens for hours and I just lie there. That's when I really shut down.

▶ **Are you aroused?**
I have an erection most of the time.

▶ **Does it bother you that you can't reach it?**
I've given up all physical control, so it's important for me to be unable to reach it. But otherwise it feels nice, like having a boner just as you're falling asleep. I call it my falling-asleep-boner.

▶ **Do you fall asleep when you're just lying there?**
Sometimes, but that is always positive. Of course, I fantasize about spending the entire night like that, but I haven't been able to do it so far. I don't really know whether it would be that much fun.

▶ **How long did your longest session last?**
Six hours.

▶ **What do you do for six hours in a bag?**
There's a lot going on in your head. All it takes is a noise, and right away a movie starts up in my head.

▶ **So, it's important for you to know you're not alone?**
Yes. "Alone but not lonely" is my motto. That doesn't mean my partner

has to look after me the whole time, it's enough for him to be there. Even if we're in different rooms, it gives me a feeling of mental and emotional connection. Otherwise I'm practically switched off and my partner has access to me any time he wants.

▶ **Like a piece of furniture?**
Something like that. Of course, if nothing happens at all for a long time, it can get kind of boring. I need stimulation from time to time.

▶ **What kind of stimulation?**
When you're closed off like that, you're very receptive. Blowing on exposed skin is enough to make my head explode. Or hearing footsteps and asking myself what might be about to happen.

▶ **Do you ever orgasm?**
(Laughs) Ever? Usually several times per session. Depends on how I'm made to ejaculate.

▶ **So, your dick is always accessible?**
It depends, but yes, usually.

▶ **So, you don't ejaculate just by hanging around?**
No. I need some action after a while.

▶ **And once it's over?**
I feel reborn. For me, it's like refueling with pure energy.

always an important factor. The duration depends on how he feels. Once pain or numbness sets in, he won't be able to relax, so you need to take the type of bondage and the position into account when deciding on what particular state you want to reach.

As with every practice, bondage is not a competition: Immobilization should only be taken as far as it corresponds to your own pleasure. In an interview with an expert, we are treated to some insights into the body and emotional world of a man who likes to "go all the way" to total mummification.

▼ Confidence and Empathy

Even if you have previously communicated the direction you want to move in sexually with your partner, whether via chat, or in a conversation or using other signals, there is always a gray zone that can be full of surprises. I don't think you can ever reach a state where you know everything about yourself, to say nothing of another man. Only if you can read between the lines, or if you meet someone who can, will sex turn in to something that knocks you off your feet (in a good way).

Now I'm skating on thin ice here, because this involves your brain—which is, after all, the largest sexual organ in men as well, whatever jokes you might have heard to the contrary. Of course, you can run through the whole program on auto-pilot—fucking, licking, blowing, getting out the toys, sticking them in, tying him up, and whipping him—but you won't enjoy it much if your partner doesn't join in. Unless he's the inflatable kind.

Good sex also involves a combination of empathy and selfishness.

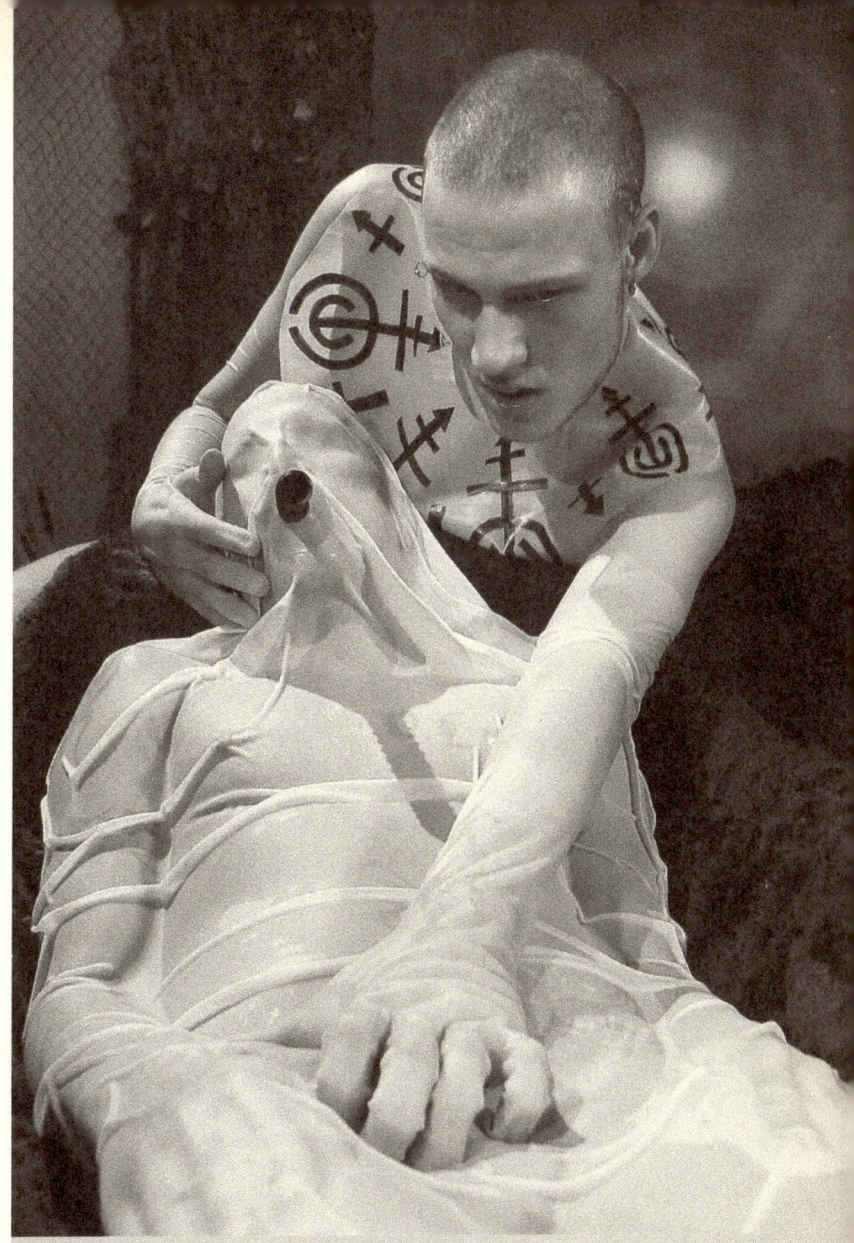

If you like it tight, you can always smooth out the wrinkles by hand.

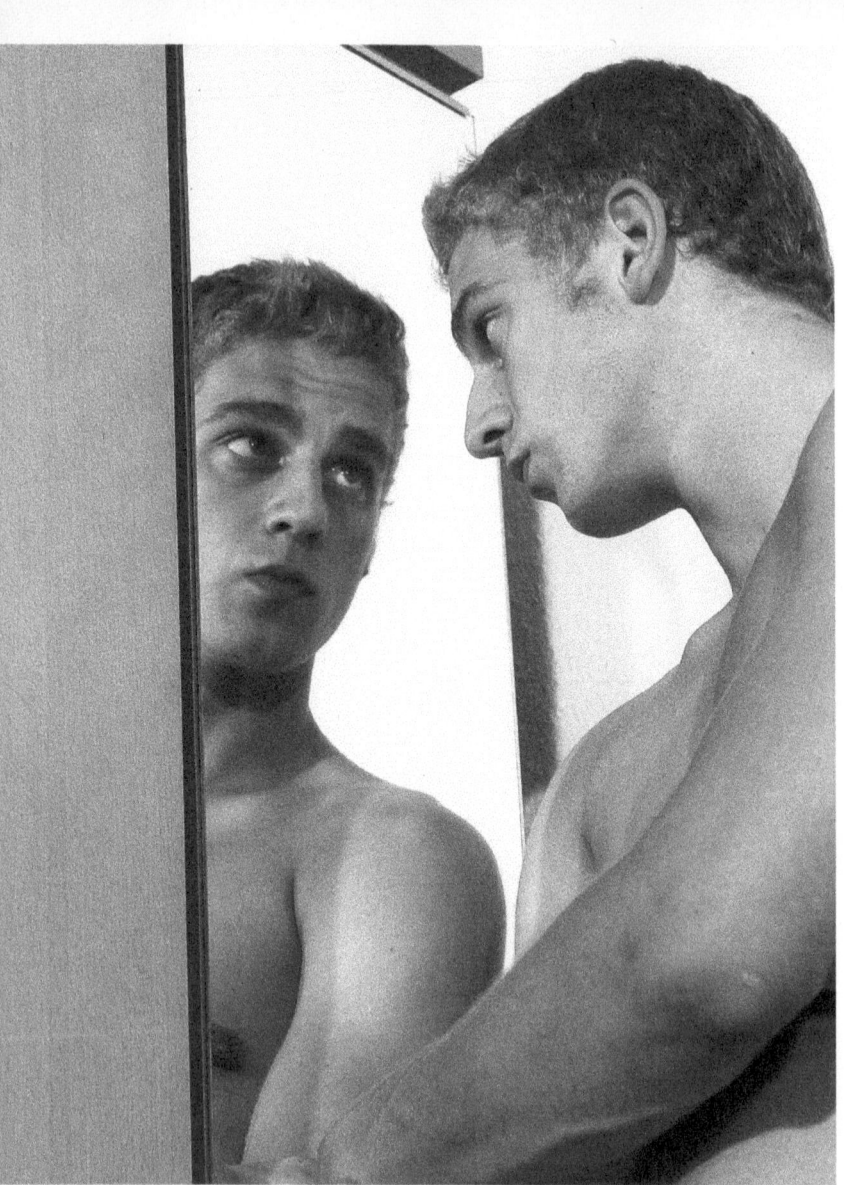

"Have we met?"

Empathy is probably the more difficult part. Even the greatest levels of expertise won't guarantee success. This is true for your professional life as much as your sex life. Your physical skills are also just one aspect of your sexuality. It doesn't matter what tricks you can do. Soft skills play an equally significant role. These include attributes such as discipline, manners, politeness, friendliness, motivation, communication skills, independence, and the ability to work in a team, but also a sense of responsibility, courage, assertiveness, and the ability to solve conflicts. These are attributes you have to learn from experience. Book learning won't help you.

That they all play some role during sex goes without saying, as this always involves two human beings interacting, both of whom have a highly individual combination of these features. Even if you meet someone in a darkroom, there are certain forms of etiquette that can have a decisive influence on your sex life. Bad behavior won't get you very far.

The extent of your capacity for empathy, another soft skill, may be crucial to your sex life and how you experience it. Empathy is the ability to understand another person as a whole, to understand his feelings as well as his emotional and other reactions. The point is not to turn yourself into the other person, but rather to objectively observe and understand him from some distance at first, which will help you to gain a clearer understanding of his opinions and actions. You have to suspend judgment of the person you are observing, it's all about understanding why he does and thinks certain things. Recognizing what values and norms are important to him and putting yourself in his shoes, even if you don't share his point of view, will allow you to detect his sexual desires. He might like whatever you do or plan to do or he might not, so an accurate assessment on your part is important, so that everything can get off to a good start.

Paying attention to signals is good practice. The clearer your signals are, the easier it will be for your partner to understand you. We have already discussed this in our chapter on "Signals." How you

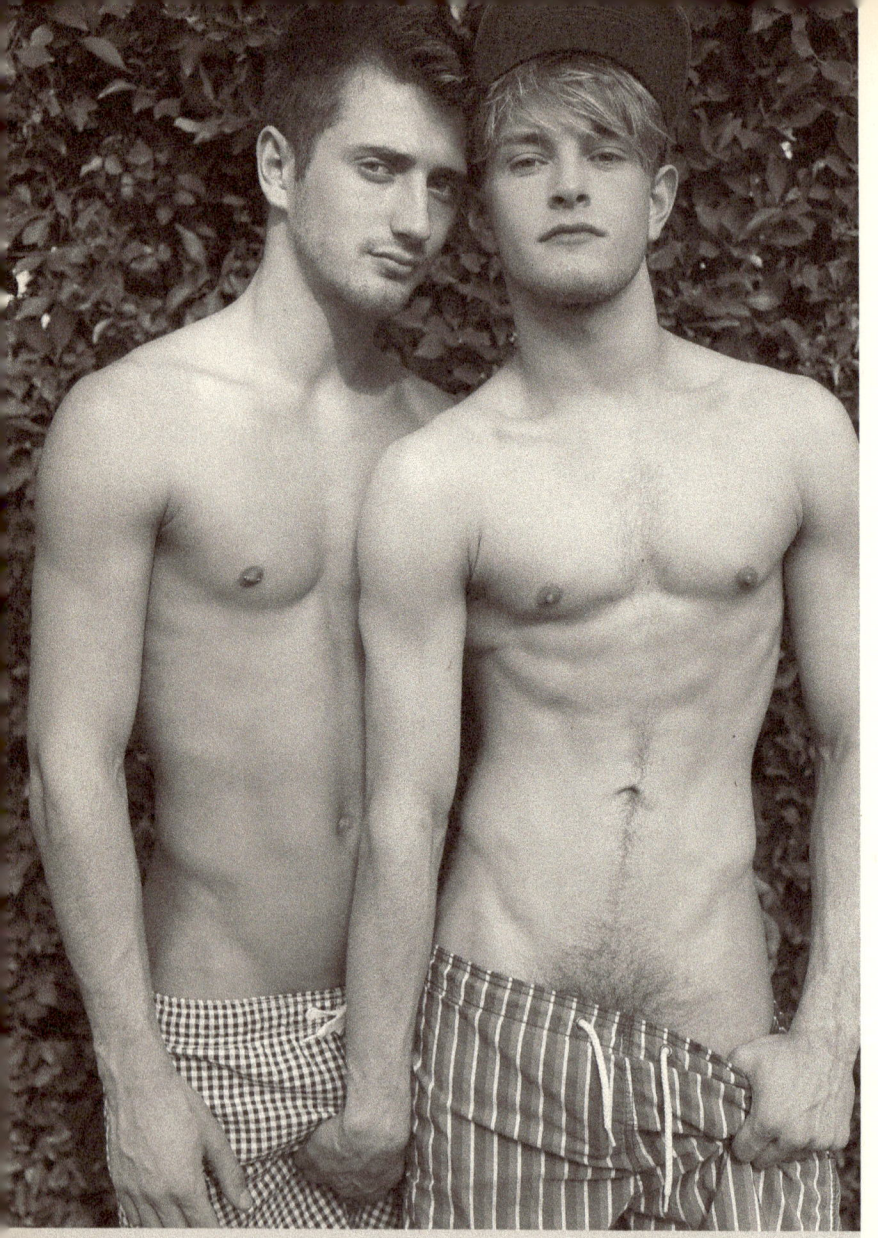

Grabbing your crotch is a sure sign that he's interested.

use them depends on you, and how to interpret them is a matter of experience. This takes practice, because signals aren't always clear. Your reactions to them will only be correct once you have understood the person behind them. Good listening skills and the ability to read body language won't come amiss in everyday life and they will enhance your ability to put yourself in another man's position.

This will also pay off in your sex life. Does your partner tell you stories about a schoolyard fight he had as a boy because he wants to try a bit of roughhousing with you, or he does he detest physical displays of strength? After looking into your eyes, does he always take a sip of his beer at the same time as you? How can you motivate him to do what you want to do sexually? The more attention you pay your partner, the better you will learn to read his signals. Even thinking about it takes a bit of empathy.

A good way of getting attuned to your partner during sex is to breathe together. In order to synchronize your rhythms, both partners have to coordinate their physical and emotional state. Breathing fast together if you're both intensely aroused—and slowly if you're relaxed and enjoying yourselves—will almost automatically create a connection between you and the other man.

▷ Just Go for It?

Thinking about the other guy's feelings, empathizing with him—sounds like work. Don't we all get off on those selfish and inconsiderate assholes that confidently fuck their way through life without so much as a backward glance? In the long term, however, the pure egotist who rides off into the sunset once he's had his way with you, is not that much fun, a really self-confident man is a better alternative. He knows that he'll get more out of it if the other guy gets something out of it, too. That's why he can and will adapt his needs to those of his partner.

Lest there be a misunderstanding: A certain amount of underhandedness in bed can never hurt. It can even be sexy, as too much compassion can prevent you from forcing the other guy to explore his own boundaries, leaving behind the stale taste of dissatisfaction. Initiating anything takes self-confidence and courage, but there you are: No risk, no fun! If you know what you want, if you think you've found the right person for it because he's sent out the right signals, then go right ahead! Your insecurity can affect the other person, that's why it's important for you to learn to deal with rejection. But unlike an egotist, a confident man doesn't rape his partner—he convinces him, carries him along. He will always be a gentleman. That's why the soft skills you need are so crucial to good sex. Finding out what fantasies you both have in common and acting on them—that takes empathy and other soft skills, but it will take you on an exciting journey into the land of sexual adventure.

▼ Voyeurism and Exhibitionism

"There's nothing better than watching two men having sex!" said a friend of mine with a happy sigh, while smoking a cigarette and watching the small orgy going on around him. I can only agree. Never a truer word was said. I'm not a creeper, but if offered the opportunity, I'm happy to be a voyeur. Of course, there is also something voyeuristic in watching a porno on DVD, but watching the live action unfold in front of you is incomparably better. "After all, voyeurism is participation!" says a quote from one of my favorite movies, *Shortbus*.

And it's true! But it also requires an exhibitionist player, someone who is aware of being watched and enjoys it, otherwise you're just a creeper. It's not always just about sex, otherwise a show like *Big Brother* wouldn't have been such a success. A somewhat nicer version of the same is a Finnish TV program aired at night. You can spend hours watching casted actors doing stuff at home on their own, stuff that ordinary people do all the time, only it's scripted.

They bake bread, eat, use the phone, etc. The show has incredible ratings, even though there's no sex. That would probably be the next step, as successfully represented on numerous Internet sites.

But in my opinion, voyeurism and exhibitionism are positive elements. They are only of interest if you are looking for something to compare with yourself, to find out who and what you are. Not being an anarchist, this makes sense to me. It's astonishing how far you can go in the relatively liberal parts of this world of ours, without renouncing your own personality. The boundaries are completely acceptable. This becomes clear when you observe other people's behavior, for instance watching two men have sex. An interest in the intimate actions of other people is probably an interest in oneself, in the broadest sense. Does the fascination, what the private or even intimate acts of another person hold for us, stem from our search for ourselves?

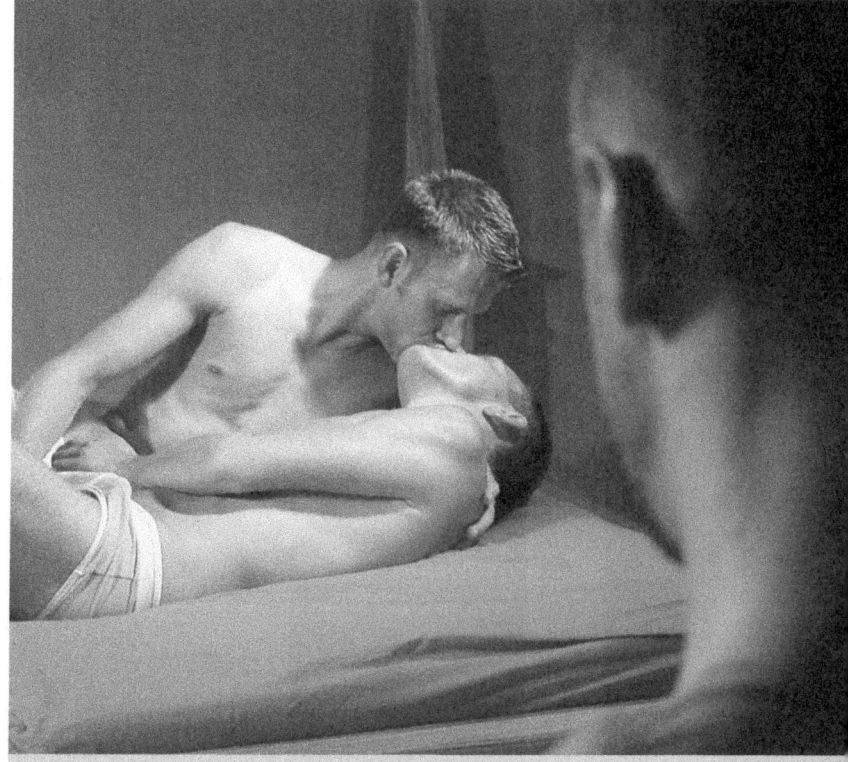

He didn't know if he'd rather be a cameraman or a director.

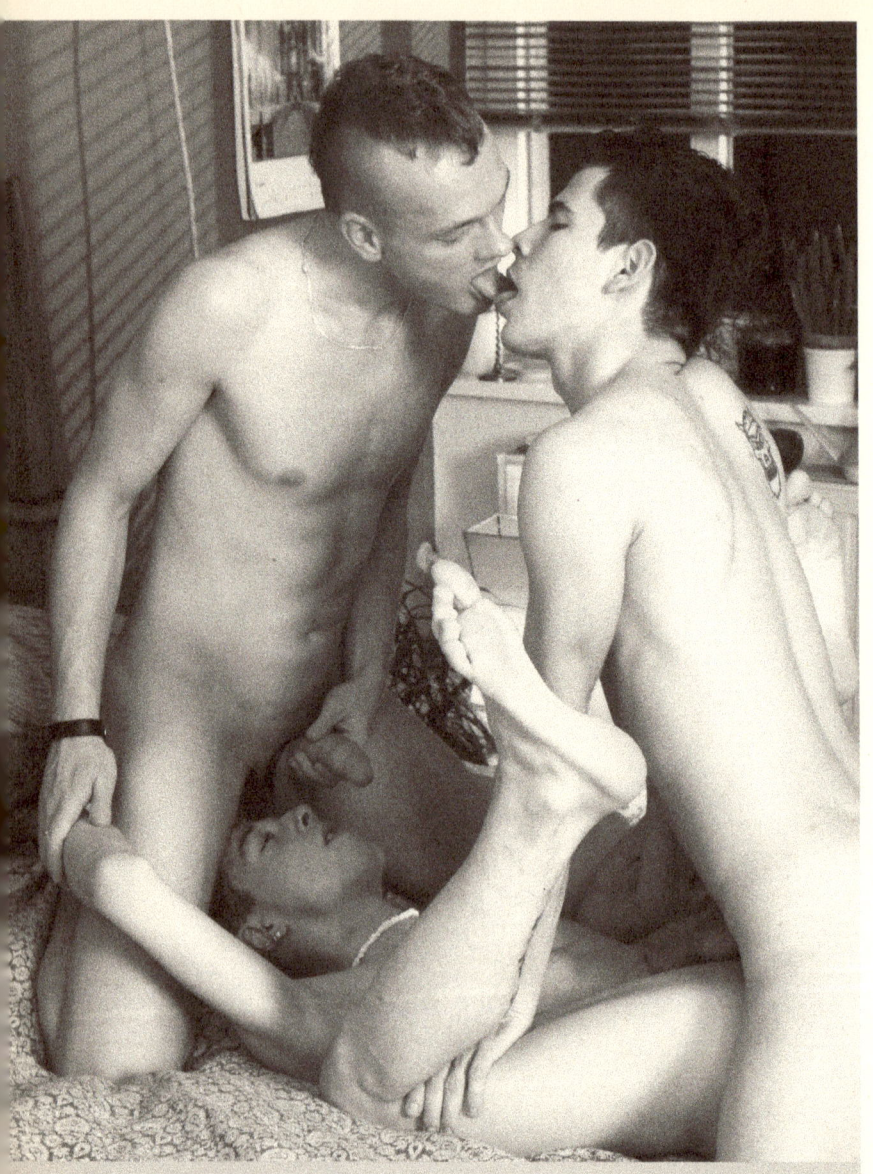

There's always room for one more.

Live Show—Sex Story with a Foursome

Brad and Corey had accepted Bruce and Joaquin's invitation and immediately felt right at home with these two hot guys. They had been carrying on with each other in turn for over an hour already. Corey was just taking a break on the recliner. He watched as his boyfriend fucked Joaquin in the sling. Bruce lay under the sling and was treated to the view of Brad shoving his thick rod into Joaquin's ass. He knew what Brad must be feeling, as his own dick had been rammed into the same hole shortly beforehand. Joaquin's muscular tube had closed around his shaft, as soft as butter, massaging it, just as it was presumably doing now to Brad's cock.

His assumptions were confirmed by a low moan from Brad. *Leave it to Joaquin!* he said to himself and grinned as he watched his boyfriend getting pounded. After a while he'd had enough of genitals for the moment. Now he wanted to see some happy faces! He drew his wet tongue over Brad's balls and through his crack from below and stood up next to the sling. Brad stroked Joaquin's sweaty chest as he fucked him and stared deep into his eyes. Bruce could feel the passion between the two guys and it made him happy. He beat off almost mechanically. Joaquin turned his opened mouth towards him.

Bruce was aware of Brad's eyes following him, waiting for what would happen next. This turned him on. He let his dick play around the parted lips that longed to suck on it. He pressed the glans against them and pulled it away again before they could close on it. No matter how Joaquin snatched at it, Bruce teased him, keeping it out of his reach. As Joaquin's greed visibly increased, Bruce threw a glance at Brad and they exchanged an evil grin. This was hot! Joaquin finally had his way as Bruce stuffed his thick cock into his mouth. Closing his eyes, Bruce enjoyed the sensation of his boyfriend's soft sucking mouth, while Brad stuffed the other hole. Brad loved the sight of Joaquin swallowing the long shaft from the glans to the root, again and again. He felt the pulsating heat around his own dick, deep inside Joaquin. The awareness of the circuit that connected the three of them kicked into his spinal cord. He thrust harder. And again.

Joaquin interrupted his sucking to throw a brief glance at Brad, whose glittering eyes confirmed how turned on he was. He was totally happy with the somewhat rougher play. The room was suffused with the smell of lust and sweat.

The two guys slapped noisily into each other with each thrust. This animated Corey in the recliner to rejoin the group. Stroking his dick, he approached the other three, stood behind his boyfriend and embraced him. He pressed against the sweaty male body and felt the force with which Brad was ramming his thick cock into the willing hole of the guy in the sling. A glance over his shoulder and he could see the thick shaft going in and out of the damp orifice. Corey passed his hand through his boyfriend's legs, grabbed his swollen balls and felt for the stretch in the fucked hole by pushing one, and then two fingers in past the throbbing shaft, deep into the slippery hotness.

Joaquin moaned in his sling. The added stimulation of the fingers moving in his ass made him feel as if the dick inside him had grown even thicker. Then suddenly they slipped out again, leaving him with the feeling of the pounding shaft that went on fucking him.

Corey went around the sling and stood at the head, where Joaquin was still pleasuring Bruce's knob with his mouth. For a while, he watched as the tongue and lips played with the damp smooth tip, before the thick muscular shaft disappeared far into his throat. Joaquin had a beautiful mouth, with soft fleshy lips. Corey placed his cock next to Bruce's darker dick and Joaquin's warm tongue immediately began to lap around both the tips, mingling their juices. Joaquin smiled beatifically like a small boy happily licking two ice cream cones.

Corey shot Bruce a grin. If this went on, Joaquin was next in line for a double helping of cream—that much was clear!

Bruce had another idea.

"Open wide!" he commanded his boyfriend in the sling. Joaquin immediately obeyed and panted with his mouth wide open. Corey watched as Bruce spat into the other man's mouth a couple of times. A white gob of spit hung from his nose and chin and Joaquin greedily tried to reach it with the tip of his tongue. Hot! Corey felt like trying it himself.

"Open up!" he said. In an instant, Joaquin turned to him and opened his mouth wide. He appeared to be well trained. There would no doubt be further opportunities for testing his obedience. Corey let a string of spittle dangle down, which Joaquin caught with enthusiasm. Then he winked at his boyfriend Brad, who had been watching him in between thrusts. Brad grinned at him: Yes, this command-and-obey game was a real turn-on! Maybe they could do it again sometime?

▼ Dominant or Submissive?

The terms active/passive and dominant/submissive don't always need to be clearly applied to one person. Not even in the strictly regulated world of S&M. A good "master" will always be attuned to his "slave," which means he submits as well. A passive slut can actively demand acceptance of his services. As most men have each component within them—sometimes more, sometimes less highly developed—a number of hybrid forms are possible. Special terms are used in an attempt to clarify, especially in S&M. The dominant partner can be called a "dom," a "top," a "dom top," or "master," the submissive partner is a "sub," "bottom," or "slave."

Men generally take well to finding their own place within a hierarchy. Even boys are great fans of hierarchical structures, as any group game will soon show. They willingly see their actions as part of a larger collective as long as it is clear who makes the rules and as long as the rules are applied fairly. A clear allocation of roles can also play a part during sex and be enjoyable within this framework. The active partner should take on the dominant role, but that means that there has to be an "active" and a "passive" player. Being able to switch roles occasionally is a big plus for gay sex.

Among gay men, the guy doing the fucking or on the receiving end of a blow job is called active, and the guy being fucked or doing the blowing is the passive one. So allowing yourself to be penetrated is generally seen as being passive. On the other hand, very few men have a problem with being sucked off at least once in a while, whether they're active or passive. It really is the greatest, having your dick pleasured by the warm, wet mouth of another man, having him suck at it slowly and appreciatively ... Where was I? Oh right, devotion!

▶ Devotion or Submission?

Submissive men are generally characterized by their tendency to see the other guy's pleasure and satisfaction as more important than their own. They enjoy "being of service." However, wanting to give your partner pleasure is generally a given in most conventional sexual relationships between two men. As a rule, submissive/passive acts alternate with dominant/active ones. Even the act of consenting to a presumably submissive act is itself active. If consent takes place in a context where you actually reject the act but experience pleasure in your loathing of what is being done to you, this is a masochistic trait—but that is just a definition, not a judgment.

If you let your partner determine what will happen for a while, part of your enjoyment can simply be for him to take on the responsibility for what you're about to do. For this, you have to be able to trust him to a certain extent. That way you can let yourself be lead and just let it happen. Your submission should also be accepted for what it is. At best, it will make you feel safe and let you cast off your desire for control for a while. Forgetting your fears and just letting yourself be pampered or used can sometimes help you shake off your problems and frustrations. It can be a turn-on feeling and enjoying another man's strength without fear, submitting to his will, feeling his physical power. Every man has strength and vigor, if you give him enough space to show it. Even something as simple closing your eyes can tell your partner that you are ready for him to take the initiative.

The transition from submissive to dominant is an easy one. As soon as you have an idea of your own and would like to carry it out, you just take the lead and become the active, dominant partner.

But what about the other way around? You would like to not be dominant for a change, would like to relinquish control and let your partner decide what to do next. Of course, in that case, your partner needs to have a plan, or at least an idea. What happens now? "Should I make a move for his pants?" This idea needs to come to him first and then he has to make the decision to carry it out. If you just

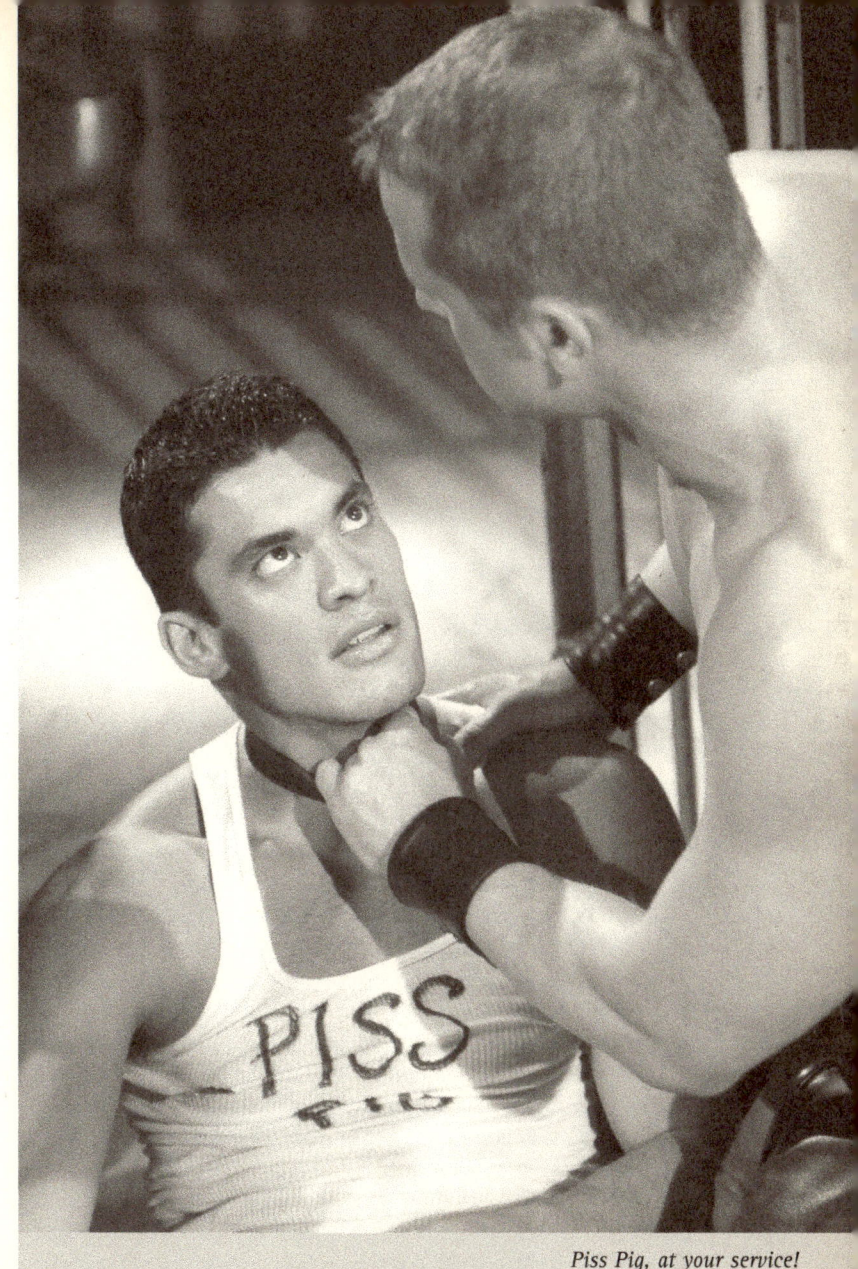

Piss Pig, at your service!

stand there, hopefully he'll come up with something. Obviously, the transition is only possible if both partners want it. That will be the case for every couple, at least once in a while. After all, every active partner would like to give up control for a while. That doesn't mean rape him! You can lead him, but that doesn't necessarily mean you can or even want to use him.

▶ Convincing or Dominant?

Playing with traditional "active" and "dominant" male roles can be especially fun during sex between two men.

If you regularly take the initiative for a longer period of time, you automatically become the active, dominant partner. You can be just as much yourself in this role as you were in the passive role just before or last time. There is a lot of speculation over the best active partners being the ones who have had experience in a passive role. This is born out by the fact that they can understand active/dominant acts. But dominance does require a certain measure of empathy. As rough and ready as some leather stallions might be, they are no good at all if they are not aware of certain reactions and signals. At least, they are no good at really good sex. Someone who just wants to sate his lust with the aid of some random assistant isn't going to carefully entice you along the path he's chosen and consciously create a space for action and experiences that may go beyond your established boundaries. Not charging on ahead, while at the same time not being too insecure—that is the true art of good sex (see also *Empathy and Selfishness* and *Movement and Standstill*). Your greatest obstacle is your own insecurity, which you have to either overcome or at least conceal. Nervous movements, absent mindedness such as ripping a rubber while you're putting it on or knocking over a bottle, can make your partner nervous, too, and ruin the whole session. But these things happen. Even an expert can have a bad day. If you can laugh at yourself in these kinds of situations, then you've found the nicest way out of the presumed mess. At the very least, don't turn it into a huge drama! As long as

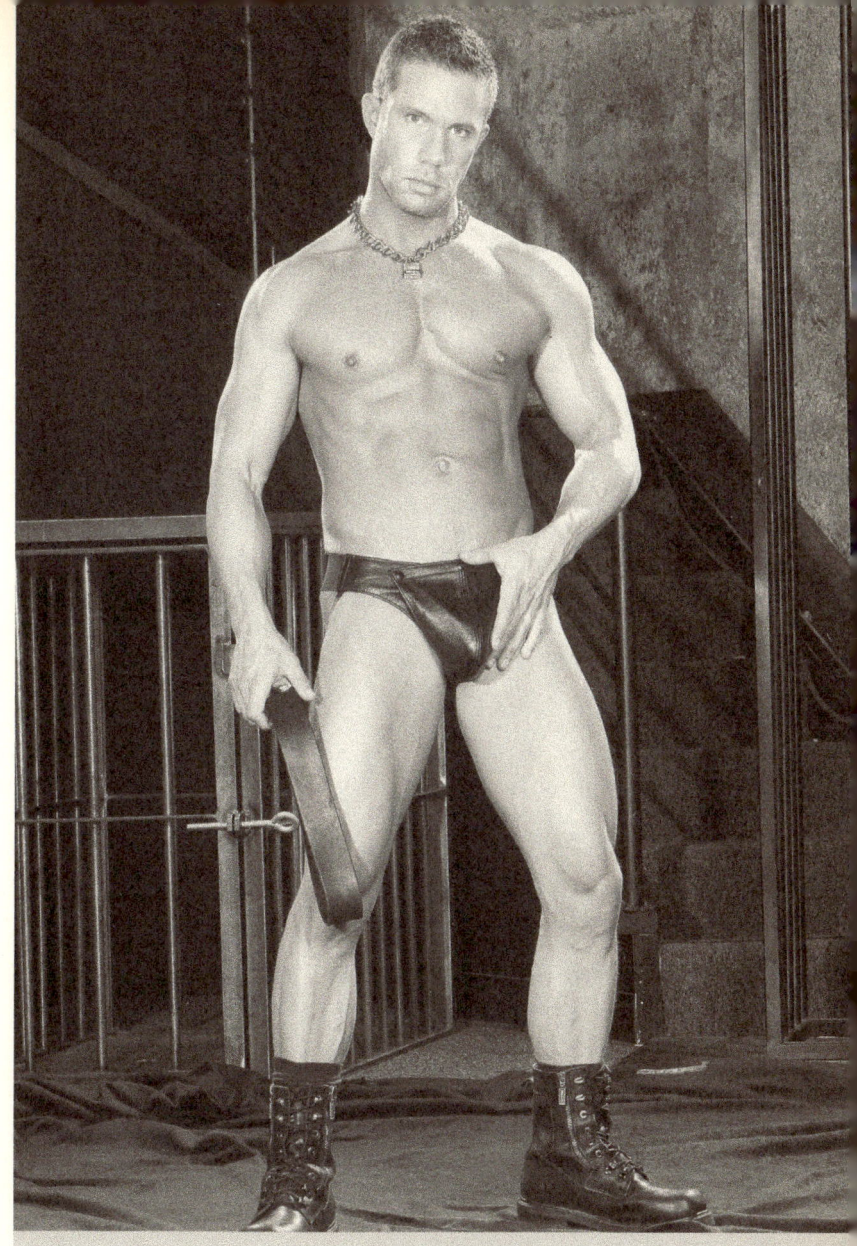

First the belt and then the mighty sword.

At His Mercy—
An Interview with Herrmeistersir

In master and slave role-play, dominance and submission are acted out to their full extent. What does it mean to be a "slave" or a "master"? Do these terms contain any usable elements that can be incorporated into a totally run-of-the-mill sexual adventure? It doesn't have to be a master/slave relationship 24-7. Being at someone else's mercy and giving up all control for twenty-four hours a day, seven days a week sounds alarming and unrealistic. But just for one night, for one session? This is not about reaching the higher orders of "real" slaves and "real" masters. How far can you take this game of self-surrender? A friend of mine has dedicated himself to the philosophy of this topic. As a recognized and respected master, he has answered a few of my questions of the subject of dominance. We are therefore talking about "BDSM." The term is made up of the first letters of bondage & discipline, dominance & submission, and sadism & masochism. So, aside from dominance and submission, bondage play, pleasure pain, and playful punishment are also part of this sexual practice. We will be taking a closer look at the topic of pain and pleasure in our next chapter.

My dear friend Herrmeistersir (HMR) lives in Seattle. Not only is he a beautiful hunk of a man, his spirit is outstanding and inspiring. He has learned a great deal about what it means to be a dom top, due to his experience with a great number of subs, slaves, and bottoms, who worshiped the dirt underneath his impressive boots, and still do. He agreed to answer some questions about tops and bottoms, domination and devotion.

▸ **What makes a top a good top, sir?**
HMR: Let's be clear. I can't speak for anyone else, because there are always exceptions within nature. (Laughs) There are plenty of tops, but few good ones. As a master sir, I think it is important to not get stuck on labels without having a healthy respect for them. There are few tops who are dominant types. Then beyond that, you have doms who are skilled masters. Nine times out of ten, the doms are tops or switches.
In my experience, masters rarely switch because their purpose is focused on the refinement of their skills and wisdom as a master. If they do switch, it is often on a limited basis with someone they find more skilled or wish to

learn from—or they simply want to experience what another does by being on the receiving end. I think for someone like me, a switch makes a good confident boy or partner in play for me to use and direct. They are only good slave material if the switching is about sexual topping or bottoming while always maintaining the heart and spirit of a slave while in the act of doing either.

I believe the best dom/masters are perceptive, imaginative, and receptive. Even a bottom can be a good top but a good dom/master, among other things, has to be a good listener and intuits much of what is going on around him. His ego has to be the beast he keeps in the cage, and when it does come out, he better make sure he has a good whip to keep it in alignment with his purpose and play.

The good dom is willing to dig down inside of the bottom to guide, arouse, and push him to new levels of awareness. The scary part that really makes a difference is the ability to sense inside of another and move around in their headspace using your verbal, breathing, touching, smelling, and listening skills. Like any good artist or craftsman, you have to feel and discern with your whole being. If you are just letting your male member do all of the work, you are a piss-poor top in my book.

In a number of cases he has, at some point in his sexual journey, been a very receptive bottom. That is the case with me. A good indicator for me as to the abilities of someone in the bed is, how comfortable are they on the dance floor? A man who is able to catch a rhythm or a beat from music that moves your hips will know how to ride rhythms and feel the beat of a bottom. If you want to learn how to be receptive, learn to take drum music in heart, abs, hips, and groins and not the head—that's analytical thinking, not dancing.

▸ **What makes a bottom a good bottom?**
He has got to be fearless. A wise daredevil. Someone who relaxes and takes his partner inside of him beyond the physical expression. Good sex is like a good dance or a massage, an exchange you have to be willing to allow yourself to get lost in.

▸ **Do you have a checklist for bottoms?**
Since my form of sexual expression is about transformation through the erotic, I tend to look a little deeper. When I meet someone, I want to know if

they are trustworthy. I want to discover what makes them unique and what scares and entices them at the same time. I guess my basics are as follows:

- What do their eyes tell me?
- How well do they know themselves?
- Can they see fun as being serious?
- Are they able to communicate and keep their word?
- How much fear do they have in regards to intimacy? Do they express an interest in the size of one's sexual member before all else? If so, I am not interested. This signals that they most likely see sex as a numbers game rather than an erotic exploration. Many guys always complain they can find a good top or dom—or bottom, for that matter—yet they fear intimacy. How curious and committed are they to real exploration, beyond just "getting off?"
- Do they take care of themselves physically, mentally, and spiritually?
- Have they done their homework on the culture of S&M/leather?
- Does a sub/bottom understand that role-play means you "play it" [your role] from a place of personal truth by taking risks, being vulnerable, pushing yourself beyond your limiting fears, and being honest through the lens of fun? In a scene, you have to be like an actor: You have to access a part of yourself that not your "self that is on the street." Be the self that wishes to feel and breathe what it means to a sub/bottom without self-judgment or condemnation.

▶ **Do you have a contract that your bottom has to sign? The common fantasy would be that punishment for a certain failure is listed. Does something like that exist for you?**
I know that contracts are something many adhere to for heightening the erotic experience. I think they are valid for short-term and long-term. My contracts need to be practical and doable. Unless it's a part of scene where corporal punishment is metered for every in fraction. I have done that ... of course, that's negotiated in advance. The funny thing is that I have a 24-7 live-in slave. My contract is real basic and easy: obedience, acceptance, service, and pleasing my domination. Since said slave lives with me, it has the benefit of learning all of my wishes, ins and outs, moods and foibles. Because I communicate what it is I wish from it and have provided my slave with my basic protocol, it manages quite well. Punishment is for play,

discipline is dealt out in order to correct bad behavior. I find both extremes rewarding because I get to test my skills. I find that non-reaction or silence can be as powerful as a slap to the groin or face. The question is: Does is the know the difference and the degrees to implement. (Evil grin)

▸ **Do you re-define your rules from time to time?**
A real good contract has to be living document that allows for transformation within the individuals and their bond. The best piece of advice I can give about contracts is to keep them simple and meaningful to you as the dom—and issues of safety and responsibility for scenes gone wrong need to be in there. They may not be legal documents, but they are documents of good faith.

▸ **Do you discuss all of this with your bottom? Or do you set up the new rules by yourself and then surprise him?**
We discuss. This is a shared journey. From the onset, the deal is that my sub/slave is my other set of eyes, ears, and feelings, so I rely on it to communicate and, therefore, I have to make space for a dialogue to happen. So we discuss based on what is working or not ... or we simply dissolve the contract or extend it in away that takes it to deeper level. A good dom is straightforward and works at being clear in his communications. Surprises need come naturally but they have to be of the sort that add to the experience and not distract from it.

▸ **Do you calibrate the level of pain—let's say, a scale of one to ten— with your bottom?**
Yes, I do. This is a healthy way of keeping both of us in touch with where we are. Pain is like any form of practice—gym, memorizing a liturgy, playing sports—in that it takes discipline, awareness, and conscious effort. For me, it's like lifting weights in the gym. If I expect to see and experience growth, I have to be willing and committed to applying five to ten pounds on a steady basis. I have to ask myself, Am I ready for twenty pounds? Or am I being a coward? Dom/sub bonds in pain play are like workout partners. We push each other while doing some self-inquiry. Besides, in a scene, I like the experience of puffing on a cigar and commanding my subject to tell me, "Where am I in the music scale?" Then I make them say, "Sir, ready, sir," and on up the scale we go until I get tired or they peak. Either way, I have to be

paying close attention to body temperature, placement of limbs, breathing, etc. BDSM/S&M/leather is not for those who are unaware or unconscious about their movements in life. The stakes are too high, and the natural high is quite memorable. That's why we do it.

There is a psychological dimension to the idea of pain exploration. This means there has to be a sense of rhythm and timing. I am like a black panther sniffing for moments when I can use it to arouse ... little by little. I know from experience that with every threshold you realize something new and delicious. As in all things, too much of a good thing can be counterproductive. So when I push, I have good strategy for allowing the experience to be process. Pain is like life—it is an unavoidable process.

When a bottom tells me, "I don't do pain," I laugh. Taking someone from the rear is painful ... How one processes that pain is the same skills one needs to process the pain in sadism. No much too soon without lubricant can ripe and tear membranes. The same applies to taking a good flogging. Remember, the tissue on one's back is tougher than the internal soft tissue. Which do you think is going to be more painful if tear it?

▶ **What about kissing? Is it an important part for you?**
Slaves I kiss on the forehead and head or back—not on the lips. Slaves deal with me because they want to be set apart from others. I find having slaves kiss my boots with deep devotion and passion while being barred from kissing my lips is far more intensely spiritual. This provides them the basic psychological boundary they require. On the other hand, I will kiss other tops or boys in a scene.

▶ **What about chastity?**
Oh, I love it. If I am not given the gift of saying when and how the sub gets to release, then I can't take him seriously. My job as a dom is to dominate and use whatever tools are available to me with wisdom. I find chastity is great instrument for adjusting a subject's ego. As with any tool, one has to know when it will be effective or just a distraction. But there is something to be said for chastity devices as decoration on smooth shaved skinned. (Laughs)

▶ **What about faithfulness for your bottom? Can he see other tops?**
Yes. I will, and I have—after I have screened the dom. I want the slave to

know it is of value to me. This means putting it on loan for a party or scene. In the same way that I lend my car to a friend—that means I am taking on the responsibility. So, I better trust the individual enough to do so. My slave is my prized possession. I expect it to be treated as such. So, I don't lend it out to people I don't know or I am not comfortable with.

▶ **Is it okay for you to have more than one bottom at the same period of time or in the same session?**
Yes. But I do it based on capacity and quality—not quantity. If two or more fits my intent in a scene, so be it. But if it doesn't serve, then it's a waste of time and energy. The principles of group dynamic and psychology applies even in a scene. So [it's about] knowing my purpose, assigning roles and tasks and getting commitments.

▶ **What if your bottom tries as hard as he can, but cannot fulfill your desire?**
I let the bottom/sub know that sometimes one has to work a little harder. Then there are times when I have build my subject up and work to instill confidence in them. I want my subject to feel meaning and fulfillment. Someone with low self-esteem is no fun and lacks creativity. I would even say they lack true devotion. So, I use my work to cultivate confidence and get them to laugh at themselves. When they shine, I shine. When a sub lets me down, they take it very hard. They want nothing more in the world than for me to know the pleasure they can provide. They know that is the only reason they are serving me. As such, I maintain proper expectations, perspective, and keep sight of their uniqueness.
So, when they fall short of my fulfillment, they know it's a lesson and an opportunity to improve. Whatever pressure I implement towards their change is given to them. If they continue to fall short, then I know I need to change my method or perspective. Or let them go. It works like a charm every time. A quality sub is very diligent and self-motivated. If a dom has one that is not, I highly suggest he does some self-inventory and then inventory the subject. Something is wrong—it is hiding. Investigate.

▶ **Is it an option that your bottom becomes proactive or takes the initiative?**
No, it's not an option except in the realm of obtaining clarification in

regards to my instructions. A skilled subject will know to how take initiative by asking, "Does sir wish something to be done?" The goal is surrender, to be the table on which a master sets is skills, the doorway through which he must walk and the mirror in which he must gaze to see himself. Therefore, a subject who takes initiative is being inconsiderate at best and an obstacle at worst. So, being as clear and direct as possible will eliminate the barrier very quickly. The best initiative for a sub is to kneel with head bowed and await direction. Offer yourself as a gift. The underlining question is, How good are you at gift giving? (Smiles)

▸ **Are part-time slaves or switchers annoying to you?**
No, they are not annoying to me. However, those are people who call themselves slaves without the slightest knowledge, passion, or respect for those committed to slavery. Personally, I don't believe in part-time slaves. You are or you are not one. One can surely be of service or in servitude to another erotically on a temporary or short-term basis. Slavery is a calling within the heart and a spiritual vocation. Does one stop calling themselves German when they travel abroad or move to another country? Not really. There is something fundamental within the self that always remains. It cannot be bargained with.
I believe there are true switchers in life. They are the erotic bisexuals. It means they sincerely love and appreciate the variety. It is my experience, most who call themselves switchers have made a comfort zone of indecision.

▸ **What hurts you emotionally as a top?**
Wow! What a question. I guess I would have to say that happens when I allow my ego to get in the way of wisdom. I have a very small margin of error, so when I screw up even in the slightest way I feel the impact on an emotional level. Then again, learning to keep my eyes on what matters, and by keeping it meaningful and fun, I allow myself to be fallible, vulnerable, and focused on life's sense of humor. I think a part of what I have discovered has been through my willingness to be vulnerable with my subjects. Of course, even in my vulnerability I have had to demonstrate levels of wisdom and judgment based on the individual's capacity. Let's face it, most people are so mesmerized by the mythology of dom-sub that they forget there are universal principles which still apply if one intends on evolving into their true nature.

▶ **Do you have a favorite way to dissolve a session, to come down and meet again as two adult men in the real world?**

Hmmm ... The question presupposes, at some point, that I had to let go of two male beings. I never really let that go. No matter the intensity. For me, being a human being—a spiritual being in matter—I was given the opportunity to hold myself and the other up within the refined light of BDSM/S&M/ leather. I get to toss and turn beliefs, taboos, social conditioning, fears, and courage around. For these are tools. Much of what I do is about shaping and clothing these tools in a way that allows both of us to see something deeper about ourselves than perhaps we were taught or told. So, when I leave for the frontier of a scene, I want be uplifting. Lyrical music, a sweet drink, hugging, caressing, feeling each others breathing and gentle talks ... in that moment, I've already discovered some new adventure to pursue.

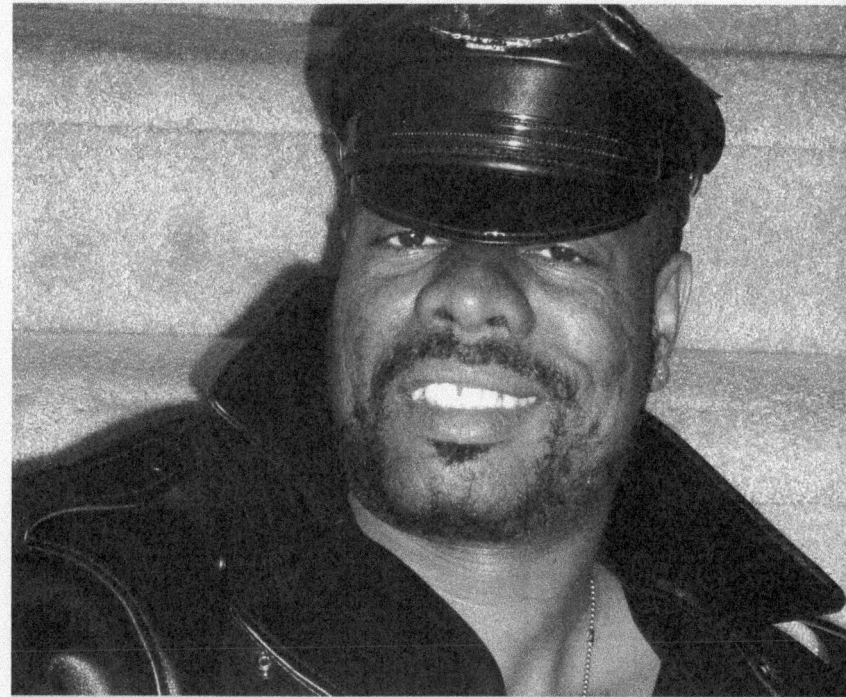

Let's all bow our heads and worship Herrmeistersir.

nothing really serious happens, I'll bet you can still motivate your partner to carry on.

If you move too quickly and it all gets to be too much for your partner, then it's up to you to deal with the situation. Of course, you can only do that if you're emotionally and physically stable enough. Being active means you need a bit of courage during sex, and there's a thin line between courage and overstepping your boundaries; most men are aware of that, so don't be afraid of making mistakes, they'll understand! Be brave!

If you do find you have ventured too far into unknown territory, it's time to backpedal. In the worst case scenario, you can just call a halt to everything and make a joke about it. You can always discuss what happened and make sure it works out next time, or you can try taking a different tack before you make your partner feel insecure.

So, the active partner always needs to have an idea of what to do next. It's easy to come up with these ideas if you put yourself in the other person's place, even if you yourself would not allow the same things to be done to you. Even if you would never let yourself be fucked/fisted/pissed on/beaten, good sex will allow for good communication between you and your partner, letting you know how he feels. It doesn't matter what means you use, whether you use words, looks, sounds or body language, communication is always an important factor.

Especially when the dominant partner gets close to a boundary—perhaps for the first time. Holding him down, grabbing his balls, covering his eyes—every action that restricts his senses or freedom of movement, requires your partner's explicit consent. Then you can go ahead and enjoy his submission!

You don't think you have it in you to be dominant? Both roles, dominant or submissive, are more fun if you are aware of your own personality. If you know who you are, you can switch roles from time to time and feel confident in your own role and with that of your partner. Really hot interactions are only possible if both partners know that they are dependent on each other for everything to work out. There has to be a top and a bottom, a certain amount of give and take. A role is right for you as long as you feel comfortable with it. No role is better or worse than the others.

Aren't dominance and submission part of every sexual interaction between two men?

▶ Role-Play

If you like to play around during sex, you might want to try slipping into a different role. Unlike on Halloween, the costumes—if there are any—are meant to be taken seriously, otherwise it's no fun. The Green Berets, who simulate a soldierly community, skinheads, leather daddies—there are all kinds of gear that point in a certain direction and can determine certain role-based behavior. Making out on a construction site while dressed up as construction workers? It's illegal, but it can be done. That doesn't mean you have to sit around in a construction crane and juggle tons of iron girders about the place. You're not going to schlep bags of cement around, either. The mere idea of: "Yes, now we're two really hot construction workers messing around with each other in the middle of the night" may already be enough. If necessary, you can heighten your awareness of the fantasy by uttering it aloud: "Yes, now we're two really hot construction workers messing around with each other in the middle of the night!"

Seducing a straight stud, being the kind of slut who lets anyone fuck him, two brothers, father and son, master and slave, (gym) teacher and pupil—these are just a few examples of typical role-play that you can follow without even needing a costume, and that will always be entertaining. Whether or not they turn you on depends on how convincing the actors are and whether or not they are able to make them work. One of the partners can be the driving force in these games by suggesting the roles, picking up the idea and creating a framework,

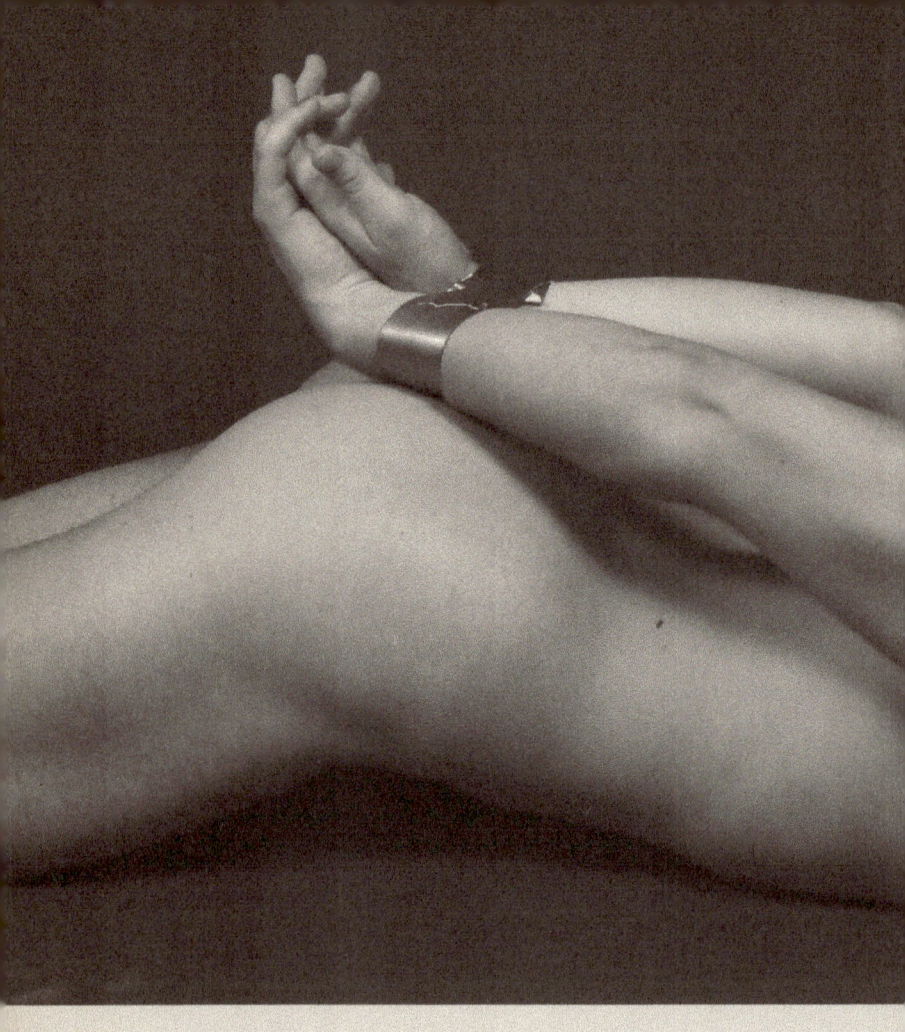

perhaps by starting out with an introductory story. Then it's generally enough to take the other guy along for the ride. Even if he's not
the world's greatest actor, he can still have fun as a bit-part player,
as long as he lets himself in for the game and is basically OK with
his allotted role. Pretending to be someone else for a short time may
strike you as rather childish at first. But you do have to be serious

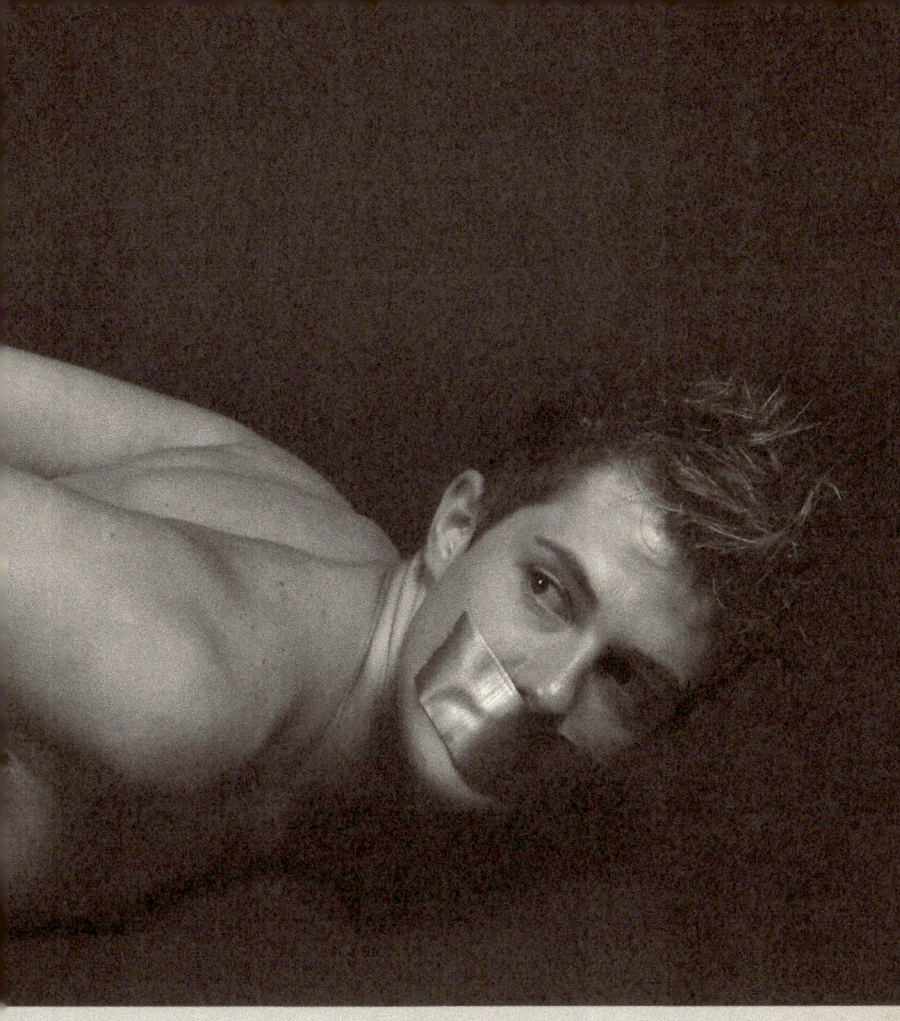

"I'll do whatever you say—just please hurt me!"

about it, because even if all you do is giggle, the whole session may still be a fun way of passing the time, but you'll never get close to diving into exciting new realms of passion. It takes courage and the will to push reality away and get into your new role during a sexual encounter. Of course, this always works best if you have the time to gradually feel your way into it. Then it can be a real turn-on to try out a different facet of male roles from the one you generally play when you're having sex.

Of course, the role needs to be a good fit. There was a time when I spied a large number of loincloths in the gay bars, and even the occasional gladiator's skirt here and there. But neither *The Jungle Book* nor the Roman fantasy seems to have found a large following.

It's a pity there are no sex parties where the roles are allocated by throwing a dice. That would be a great way to get started, either by participating or watching. You go there on your own or with a partner and then everyone is assigned a role.

And then you try it out—in public or in a private room. There are so many gay actors who would probably have the time ... or why not try it out together in your own apartment? Give me a dice! No! Not the Indian again!

Social Studies—Fifth Softcore Sex Story with Brad and Corey

After the waiter had brought them their espresso and grappa, Brad passed a card across the table.

"That doesn't look like your credit card! Why don't you give it to me?" Corey joked. He picked up the card and took a closer look.

"Motel 6," he read aloud. He grinned in amusement, but Brad's expression remained serious.

"It's just around the corner!" he said. "It's not bad. I've booked a room for us there for tonight. I've already dropped off some of our stuff."

"Great! Then let's drink up and go!" Corey was delighted.

"I'd rather you went first." Corey could see a familiar twinkle in Brad's eyes. "Why?" he asked suspiciously.

"I thought I'd get myself a rent boy tonight!" Brad answered with a wink.

"You've booked a rent boy to come up to our room?" was Corey's first thought.

"*You* can be my rent boy. A really sleazy, dirty little whore!" Brad clarified.

"Can you even afford me?" Corey tried to joke. But Brad wasn't biting.

"You're just a trashy hustler, not a luxury call boy. A couple of dollars should be enough for a cheap whore!" Brad said in defense of his low funds.

Corey realized Brad was being serious. But that was a pretty hot idea! He decided to play along.

"OK, fine—I'm your Romanian rent boy and we've arranged a date at—" he looked at his watch— "ten thirty in room twenty-five. I don't speak English and I don't understand it either."

Anticipation gave Brad a hard-on. Corey, with his dark hair and brown eyes, could be anything really, so why not Romanian?

"Great!" he agreed immediately. "I want you naked when I get there. And lubed right up!" he added.

"You pig!" Corey grinned, stood up and took the key card.

"Hey!" Brad called him back. Corey looked at his quizzically.

"What's your name?" Brad asked.

"Dushan," Corey replied. He hadn't needed to think about it. It was the name of a boy who'd once done an internship at his company.

Then he left.

Brad was unable to relax and enjoy the remaining half as much as would have liked. He ordered another grappa and repeatedly felt for the chub in his pants. He was looking forward to the hot slut waiting for him in his hotel room ...

The door opened when he knocked. He could make out the silhouette of the naked rent boy outlined against the reddish glow of the bedside lamp. "Hi!" he mumbled, then went on ahead and sat down on the edge of the bed. Nice ass!

Brad took off his jacket and placed a fifty dollar bill on the bedside table.

"Including kissing!" he demanded. The rent boy threw him a questioning look. Brad went to the bed, stroked the boy's head and leaned in for a kiss. After a brief hesitation, the rent boy's mouth opened and his tongue darted out. Not bad!

His dick pushed urgently against his fly. Brad opened his pants and tapped the tip of it a couple of times against the rent boy's fleshy lips. "Go on, take it in your mouth!" Brad commanded. "Show me you're worth the money!"

After a brief, almost arrogant glance, the hustler grabbed Brad's swollen cock and flicked his tongue over the glans before pushing his velvety lips over it. After a couple of tries, the thing had nearly reached his tonsils.

"You're pretty good!" Brad growled and stroked the cocksucker's head.

"So how many dicks have you had today?" he asked. The boy went on sucking and smiled up at him. There was no reply, he probably hadn't understood the question.

"Ten? Twenty? Thirty?" Brad wanted to know, and thrust deeper into the guy's throat with every question. The rent boy gasped and gagged.

Brad pulled him up, kissed him, and grabbed his buttocks. Turned on by the light fuzz on the cheeks, he felt for the crack. The hole was warm and slippery, a real slut's hole!

Brad was already looking forward to fucking him. He turned the hustler around, made him kneel down in front of the bed, and spread his legs. The little slut in front of him raised his tasty ass, ready to earn his fee.

Brad was in no hurry—an hour or even two would pass by quickly with this hot piece of ass!

▼ Pleasure and Pain

Nothing but tender stroking? Only gentle touching? Good sex is different, it can be hard and intense, even painful.

Sex and pain—that sounds unpleasant, that doesn't fit. Pleasure and pain, that might be a bit more familiar. In a lot of philosophical models, those are the only two feelings there are, no more. They are an unequal pair, but they belong together like the sun and the moon, night and day, no pain without pleasure and vice versa; the one thing cannot exist without the other.

Apart from its negative, distressful aspects, physical pain has another aspect. It's not easy for me to see pain as something positive, but it is at the very least a fascinating bodily phenomenon and sex is after all about the body. Can pain ever feel good?

I can't be the only person who liked to play with the liquid wax under the candle flame as a small boy. It feels so good when the (brief) pain goes away! The burning sensation starts out from the sensitive part of the body—the fingertip in this case—and spreads out through your entire body. At least that's what it feels like. The rush is not

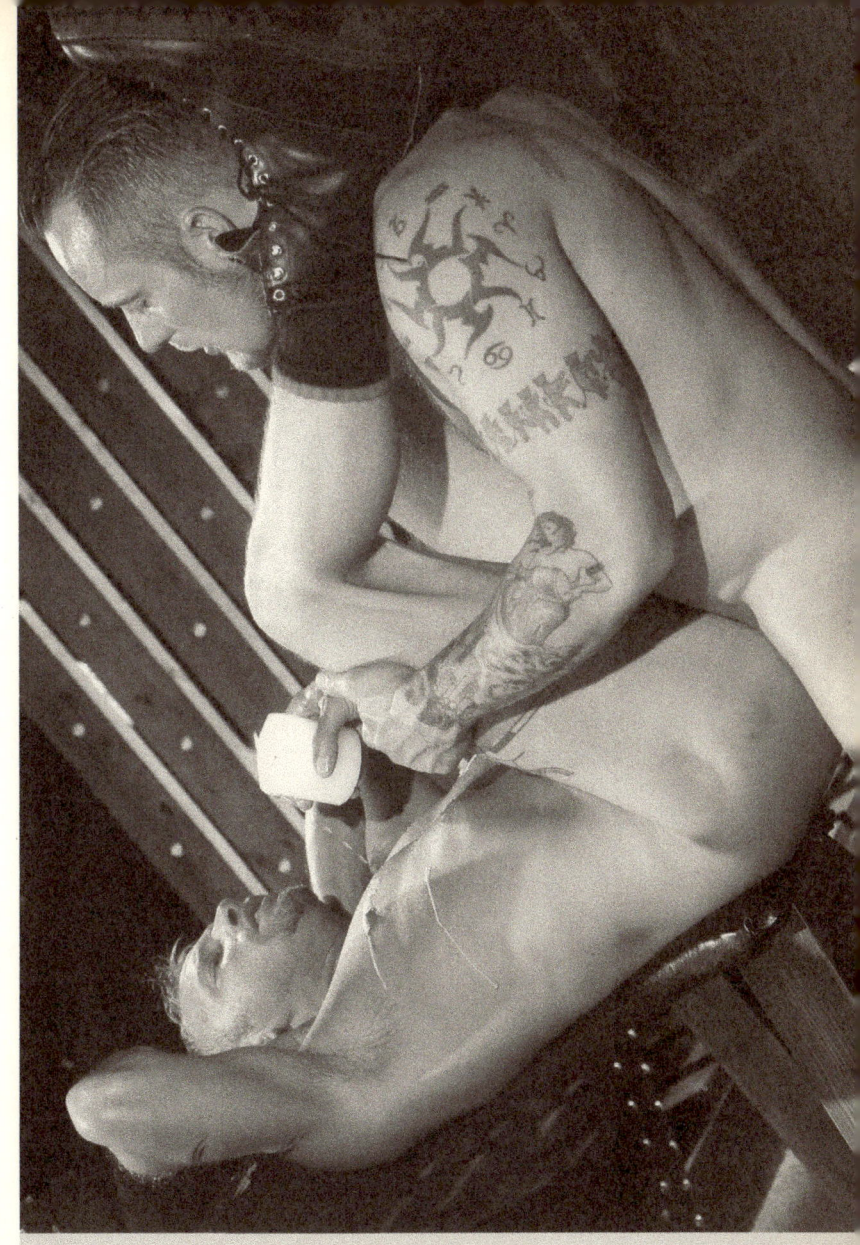

Hurts so good.

unpleasant, it's quite exciting. Pain stimulates the release of endorphins. Kissing, laughing, even working out can do the same. These neurotransmitters are commonly known as "happy hormones," and for good reason. The stronger the pain and the longer it persists, the more of them are produced by the nerve cells. Not only does this curb the pain, it can even switch it off. This effect is still subject to debate within the medical community, as is the fact that the release of endorphins can result in a feeling of happiness, even of euphoria. We are perhaps better acquainted with this state brought on by kissing, laughter, and sports. By the way, eating chili will also release an endorphin surge. The active substances in endorphins resemble those of opiates. Furthermore, endorphins are also linked to the production of sex hormones.

Happy hormones, euphoria, sex hormones—sounds OK, doesn't it?

▶ The Path of Pain

It can't hurt to know more about the pathways followed by pain within our bodies. As the pain races from the afflicted part via the spinal cord into the brain, it bears a strong resemblance to a Lady Gaga show, changing its appearance several times from start to finish. First, it is received as an impulse by the nervous system and travels along these pathways until it reaches the spinal cord. Then the pain signals are transformed into chemical transmitters. These follow the pathway of the central nervous system towards the brain. Here, the pain becomes an impulse again and penetrates out consciousness. Only then does the body react—for instance, by stimulating the production of endorphins. These latch onto your nerve cells and block the pain receptors there. By the way, testosterone is also a pain inhibitor and may be the reason why men are less sensitive to pain than women are. Despite this, women can endure pain better than men can, but that's another story.

An interesting aspect of the chain of reaction caused by pain is the connection between the nervous system and those parts of the brain responsible for emotions and emotional behavior. The nerve fibers that transmit pain run parallel to the ones that transmit feelings in your spinal cord. These two types of nervous tissue are in constant dialogue. The nerves that convey emotions send out a calming signal to the pain transmitters. The pain center in our brain is situated in the same area where our emotions are produced and where our behavior and our memories are located, namely in the limbic system, also known as the "emotional brain." So, physical pain always has an effect on our behavior and on our emotions.

Besides stimulating the production of endorphins, the mechanical action of blows and taps to the body can also release pent up energy, such as muscle tension. The increased circulation improves the removal of metabolic waste products from our tissues. These processes enhance the body's own detoxifying and regenerative mechanisms.

Another additional effect is a distinct improvement in how you perceive your body: You become more sensitive to the state and the function of individual body parts or your body as a whole.

Vulnerable areas—such as the head, neck, and the region around the heart—should, of course, be spared But apart from that, couldn't pain be another way of getting to know yourself and your body?

▷ Experiencing Pain

A gentle bite to the neck, a slap on the ass, pinching a nipple—whether or not these actions are experienced as painful depends on their context. If they are brought into play during a certain stage of desire, they are perceived differently. The more aroused you are, the more your feelings of pleasure will mask your feelings of pain. If there is more pain than pleasure, it can act as a brake. Your physical pleasure will be broken by pain, but not necessarily the pleasure in your head. That's the great thing about it. This can be a helpful way of postponing physical pleasure if you don't want all those nice feelings to get too strong and lead straight to a climax. You've probably tried this out on yourself or on a partner, consciously or unconsciously. Carefully biting your own hand at the right moment can delay orgasm. Pinching or scratching your partner's back can slow down his arousal. Repeating these or similar moves will lead to an increasing accumulation of passion, until it is finally released with heightened intensity. Pain is a more sensual method of putting the brakes on your horniness than thinking of something unpleasant—an often employed trick, despite the fact that it is a lot more strenuous, more boring, and less successful.

If you and your partner communicate well during sex and you are both aware of how aroused the other person is, it is totally OK to slow each other down and then goad each other on again. Of course, if you're in a hurry, this is counterproductive.

Otherwise, everything generally works more or less spontaneously and to a certain extent unconsciously. As a rule, our feeling for pleasure is more familiar to us than our feeling for pain, which we tend to avoid—for good reason. After all, it is a warning signal. We are most likely to inflict pain on ourselves of our own accord when working out, when our muscles start to hurt but we keep going, fighting against the pain of every fiber in our bodies. But if pain and pleasure are brothers, shouldn't we try to get to know both of them?

▷ Brotherly Pain

To set aside your pleasure for a while in order to concentrate on the interplay of pain and sensation—this has absolutely nothing to do with masochism and sadism. It's not about achieving sexual gratification through pain, but rather about experiencing the reverse side of pleasure in order to more aware of your body and its sensations.

If, having already put your fingers, lips, teeth and fingernails to good use, you can tell that your partner is receptive the new sensations, you can venture further and try out other aids. Naturally, you need to stop immediately the moment your partner gives you clear indication. The famous safe word negotiated beforehand will hopefully not be needed outside of hardcore S&M, as being aware of your partner's natural reactions and staying in constant contact with him should already be a given.

We have already discussed how switching off one sense can heighten awareness of the other senses in the chapter *Master of the Senses*. Blindfolding the eyes, immobilizing the body, or even just tying the hands can promote this effect, but they can also lead to anxiety and high expectations, resulting in many an awkward situation. It is important to give your partner the time he needs to relax and trust you, especially if you have decided to inflict pain on him for the first time. Your partner's willingness to feel and endure physical pain also plays an important part. It's best to wait until you've both gotten going properly, perhaps just before shooting your load.

There it is, the first slap landing on his ass or the first drop of wax on his skin! It takes a while for the endorphins to be released. Your partner's reactions should determine the pace with which you repeat the stimulus in the same or in another place. If he tenses up, stroking him or giving him a clear order may help release the tension and prepare him for your next action. Pain is a disturbance within our mental state. It demands immediate attention, leaving no room for any other thoughts. Your partner can endure it only because he knows that it will abate at some point. This knowledge will allow him to relax and concentrate on the moment.

Any actions that can be counted—blows, drops of wax—should also be announced. "Now I'm going to whack your left ass cheek!" Experienced S&M practitioners will "calibrate the pain" by having their partners rate the pain after every blow on a scale of one to ten, one being "weak" and ten being "very strong." That way, both partners can become attuned to one another. If your first blow is so severe that it takes your partner several minutes to deal with the shock, that really isn't the best way to begin.

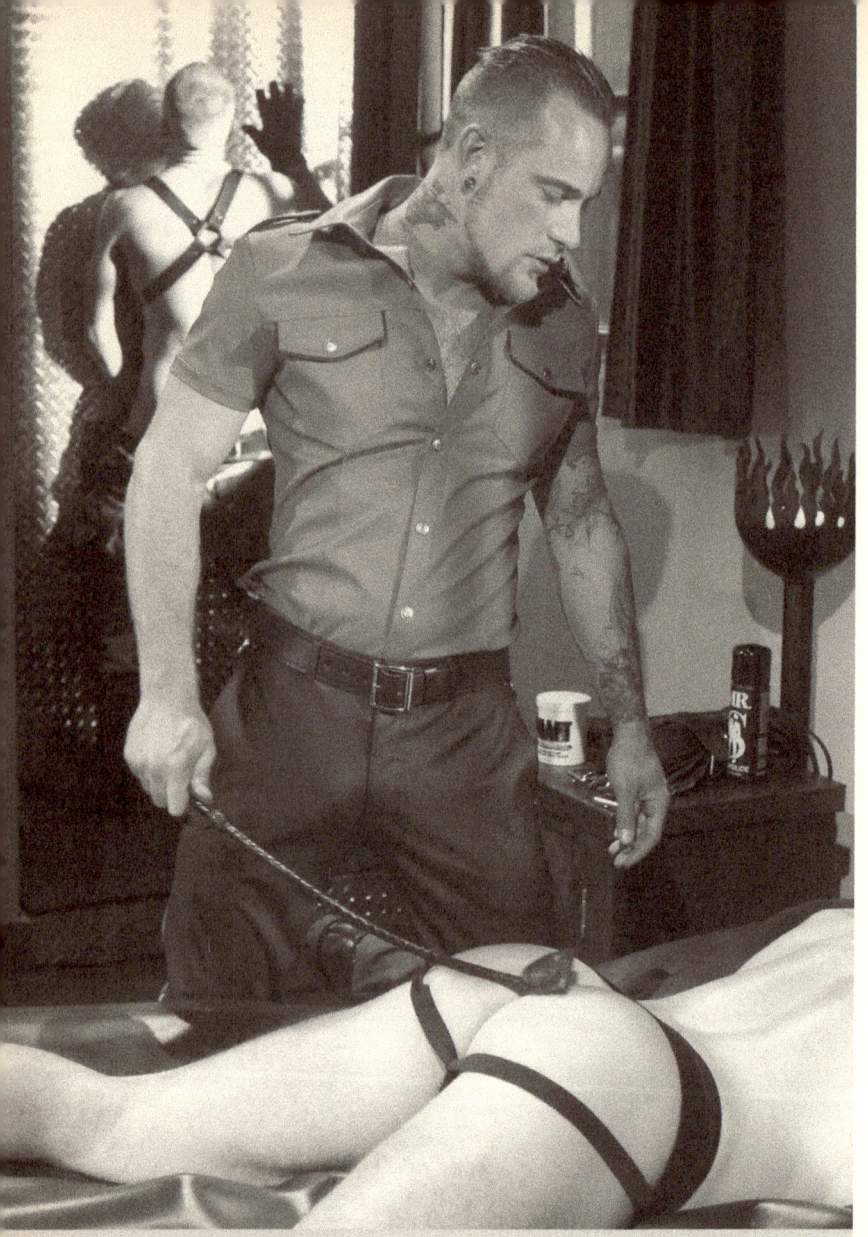

Waiting for that first blow can be painful.

Pressure, caused by clamping for instance, will inhibit circulation. The larger the clamped off area of the skin, the more the pressure will be distributed. The initial pain will abate after a time and then remain at a constant level. Please note that removing the clamps can be even more painful than attaching them, as the blood rushes back. You can do this quickly, if your partner needs to feel the pain flare up briefly, or slowly, taking time out to stroke him, if you prefer to drift along a lazier river. Perhaps a snootful of poppers would be appreciated before you remove the clamps. As we mentioned in the chapter *Scratch Me, Bite Me!* the affected area can remain sensitive and sore for hours or even days after you remove the clamp.

As we all know, the testicles are very sensitive to pain. CBT—cock and ball training—involves focusing on these delicate organs. The enormous array of cock rings you can find in sex shops just go to show the prevalence of the male penchant for paying close attention to their genitals and tying weights to them. Tying a leather strap around the scrotum, whether or not you include your dick, will increase the sensitivity of the testicles, especially if they have been individually tied off. You can control the degree of sensation, from a feeling of slight pressure to actual pain, by tying the strap more or less tightly.

Men who really get off on pain want to "ride the pain," "surf on the endorphin wave,"—they need such a high dose of pain that it makes them forget their bodies and brings on an actual high. It generally starts off with a mental ambition to be able to endure as much as possible. This lust for pain is a different kettle of fish altogether and we won't go into it here, just as we're not going to go into causing pain by cutting or pricking.

There are plenty of other ways of intentionally inflicting pain on someone without leaving visible wounds.

Any increments—more blows, more clamps—should be made in agreement with your partner. Breathing fast, sighing, or other clear signs of pleasant arousal mean that you're both on the right path.

There is no need to hurry. Stick with the same level for a while, try breathing at the same time and then gradually increase the intensity. Again, telling your partner what you're going to do is a good way of letting him adapt to whatever awaits him.

Ballgame—Fifth Hardcore Sex Story with Bruce and Joaquin

Joaquin was standing, or rather hanging, in the middle of the room, for his outstretched arms were tied to hooks in the wall to his left and right. His legs were fixed slightly apart, but Joaquin's feet were both firmly on the ground. A pair of boots dangled between his legs, tied to his balls.

Joaquin groaned quietly as he made the boots swing back and forth on the end of their leather strap. He kept his eyes closed and concentrated on the sensation. The weight tugged painlessly at his balls. The constant pull made him aware of how sensitive his testicles were, but they seemed to be doing OK. No need to worry about his crown jewels. Bruce stood in front of him. Joaquin could sense the presence of his body without looking at him. A kiss brought him back to full consciousness. He was pleased to see Bruce's relaxed face. He enjoyed surrendering himself up. Now Bruce's hand slipped over his eyes, nose, and lips, and the edge of it was shoved between his teeth up to the corners of his mouth, as if to prevent him from biting. Then Bruce drew his hand down his neck, down his chest, along his belly, and around the back. Bruce grabbed an ass cheek and squeezed the flesh, still sensitive from the blows earlier on. His hand felt hot.

With a few gentle slaps, Bruce loosened up the muscle before striking him hard. Joaquin flinched and jerked forwards, colliding with Bruce's body. Bruce grasped him tightly with his other arm. Joaquin sighed as the flash of pain became a soothing warmth. Just as his awareness was about to turn to his nuts again, the next blow followed.

Again, he concentrated on the pain in the afflicted part of his ass. Bruce knocked the dangling boots back and forth with his knee, while he held Joaquin tightly and securely. Now the pressure in his balls increased, pain rushed through the place where they were cinched together with the leather strap. Another blow in the same place, and his attention turned straight back to his ass!

They repeated this game of ping-pong a couple of times. A blow, a sigh, leaning forwards. Swinging forwards, tipping back, a sigh. Every time Bruce repeated the action, it was promptly met with the same response from Joaquin, who still managed to look surprised every time, rather than tormented. They continued this until the sheer predictability of the whole thing made them both laugh.

Bruce held Joaquin closely, stroked his heated ass cheek and kissed him passionately. Joaquin relaxed and let himself sink into Bruce's arms as far as his bonds would let him.

After a while Bruce let go of him and left the room. Joaquin rested, enjoying the burning sensation on his ass. Bruce returned shortly. In one hand, he held the spray bottle he used to spray his plants. Joaquin smiled.

He had an inkling ...

Bruce stood behind him and sprayed his heated ass with cool water. Right away, a prickling sensation started up in his ass and soon spread throughout his entire body. It gave Joaquin goose bumps.

Bruce stroked the naked body before him in fascination. "Wow!" he marveled over his partner's astonishing skin reaction. Joaquin was surprised himself, but felt almost proud, as if he had just given Bruce a gift.

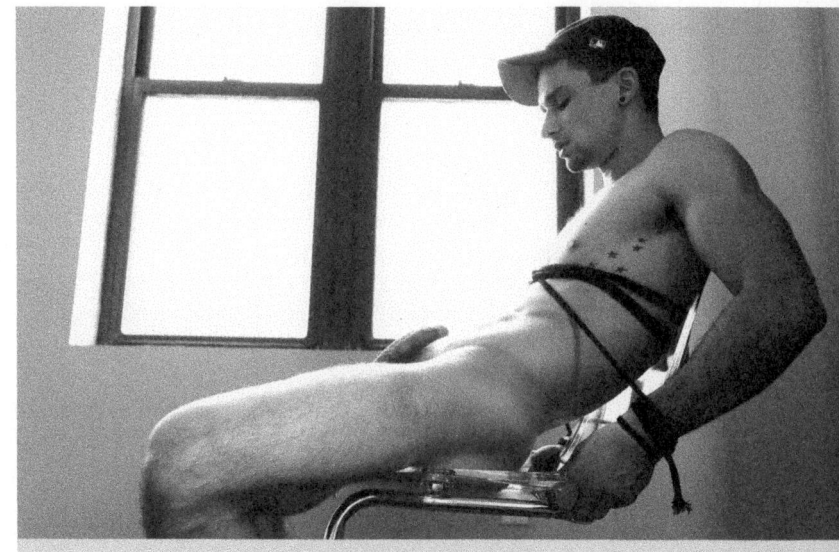

All trussed up: Let the fun begin.

Body and Soul – An Interview with Fred

Fred is forty years old, a theologian, and well known and loved throughout Munich's fetish community. Does he have any advice for us on how to steer through the wilderness of lust and desire without getting hurt?

▸ **You yourself mentioned the union of body and soul. What is the difference between a gay man who follows his desires soulfully and one who does the same with no consideration for his soul at all?**
Fred: The union of body and soul can be achieved once you experience physical gratification that also corresponds to your soul, that is to say your innermost needs. However, sexuality in the actual sense of the word means the physical union of two people. If your sexuality is directed solely towards objects, such as leather or underwear, then it is not this kind of union.

▸ **Does soulful sex have anything to do with our desire for union with another person?**
In my opinion, sex that includes both the body and the soul is the opposite of egotistical sex, which is only about the self. It is sex between two human beings enjoying each other with their bodies and with their innermost selves, where each of them is aware of their mutual responsibility for each other.

▸ **As long as that is the case, then anything goes?**
Yes, in principal. If a fetish is associated with another person or if it's a practice that requires another partner to carry it out and fulfill these needs, there has to be a certain amount of trust between both partners. For instance, in submission, pain, or BDSM practices, there are profoundly human and personal desires involved. As long as the person is still viewed as a whole and you are always aware of your responsibility for the other person, I'd say this sex does include the body and the soul. I think that the best S&M masters are generally very responsible people, with very good reason, and the know exactly what they are doing and how far they can go with whom.

▶ **So, a master who uses his slave purely for his own selfish gratification, is a bad master?**

The phenomenon of using another person, so to speak, which presumably happens quite often, especially with anonymous sex in a darkroom, can only work if it involves two people who have a need to be used or to use someone. No one will let himself be used if that's not what he wants. If it does turn out differently, it probably won't be remembered as a pleasant experience. I've heard many people tell me that they have let their own insecurity or drugs make them consent to a kind of sex that does not correspond to their true needs. They regret it afterwards.

▶ **During one of our conversations you also mentioned the biblical term of "knowing" as a term for sexual union. Does that mean being aware of the other man and knowing what he wants or doesn't want?**

Sexual acts are always an act of communication between two people who allow each other profound insights into essential aspects of their personality, namely their sexuality. They reveal desires and needs that remain hidden in everyday life and are glossed over as they represent part of our most intimate private thoughts. Revealing ourselves to our partner means that we give him the opportunity to find out more about himself than he would in everyday life and to reveal himself to us. I think that the Old Testament uses the metaphor of "knowing," to signify sexual intercourse for good reason. The fact that we experience sex with a familiar partner as qualitatively better can be traced back not only to our mutual feelings of affection, but also to the fact that we know the other man, we know his desires and needs, and we can meet these needs.

▶ **And you can't see these needs and desires in a darkroom?**

Yes, you can. You have misunderstood me. You can know another man and his deepest sexual needs, even in a darkroom.

The question is, what happens next. I think a lot of us have experienced this during darkroom sex, suddenly realizing that the other man has totally different needs and that they don't fit together at all. So, you call the whole thing off, otherwise you won't be able to have sex with your body and soul? If you realize that the other man just wants to cuddle and stroke you tenderly, for example, because he's looking for security, and you can't or won't give it to him, then yes. Or if your darkroom partner should become aggressive and violent and that's not what you want, or if he just wants you to wait on him because he's only concerned for himself.

▶ **Should we generally condemn any human desire to just have really hot, animal sex and not worry about the spiritual component?**
I think everyone needs to decide for himself as to whether he wants to switch off his mind, which is what makes him human and sets him apart from the animals. For only in this case would I say that this is animal sex in the proper sense of the word. But generally when we talk about animal sex, we mean wild, uninhibited sex, where we don't think much. But I think it would be irresponsible to completely turn off your mind and I don't think that there are many people who really want sex with no boundaries at all. Or can anyone really say he'd like it if his partner bit his penis in a fit of wild animal passion, or went on thoughtlessly fucking him, even though he's already bleeding?

▶ **How far can you take a healthy gratification of desire without damaging your own personal and spiritual integrity?**
Sexuality is a basic human need, and so gratifying it is, of course, healthy. Suppressing human needs usually causes psychological damage. This gratification will be healthy as long as it isn't used to compensate for personal shortcomings, for example, if it's the only kind of success you every have in life. The danger of becoming addicted to sex is a very real one in these cases.

▶ **Is there a universally applicable warning system, or do you just use your personal guilty or guilt-free conscience as a standard?**
I'm afraid there is no such thing as a generally applicable warning system,

because that would require an awareness of yourself and self-contemplation, and that depends on your mind and degree of intelligence, which isn't the same for everyone. But just using your conscience as a standard would mean excusing everyone's bad behavior.

▶ **What advice would you give gay men concerning their sexuality to make sure they can go through life with honor and integrity?**
I think that gay men need to be careful not to define themselves only by their sexuality. Your sexuality is an important part of your personality, but it's not the only part. Homosexuality should be lived sensibly and respectfully, and ideally in deep affection for another man—in other words, love! But it should not become the center of your existence and day-to-day life. This can lead to a dependency you won't be able to handle as you get older. Balance and proportion are the crucial terms here. And quality rather than quantity!

▶ **How do you yourself manage to attune your own desires to your spiritual needs?**
I think that question is best answered by everything I've said so far.

▼ Between Beasts and Gods

Now that I've talked about all the gloriously dirty deeds you can do with each other, I would also like to mention the mental aspects of any sexual encounter between two (or more) men, as these are also a part of the mix if you want good sex. Talking about them is possibly even more fraught with inhibitions than talking about the physical aspects.

It's not so easy to really let yourself go during sex. You can't really relax during sex until you have accepted your body and your desires and made them part of your enjoyment. It works best if both men are into it with both body and soul. I can't be the only one to think that every time two men enjoy sex with each other, they bring peace and goodwill on earth just a little bit closer.

Our bodies may be beasts, our desires and instincts primal, but sex actually takes place in our heads, our minds. Sexuality and morals are two completely different things: One of them comes from within and the other comes from outside ourselves. Guilt, shame, and fear can ruin sex, unless they are part of psychological role-play within a given framework.

I've already discussed the essential part that mutual respect plays, no matter what the relation may be between reality and the role you're playing ("Ground Rule: Respect." "Dominant or Submissive?").

Another man is your partner in horniness, and the two of you have more in common than you might think. He has the same longing for life and passion as you—perhaps he just expresses it differently. Accepting his desire, allowing yourself to be swept along, or sweeping him along yourself, enjoying physical passion with him without remorse—this can take you into another dimension. Whether or not you are completely satisfied depends on something else.

The hunger for forgetfulness, to forget one's own dull existence, cannot be sated by any kind of sexual activity. However hard you might try to have bestial, animal sex, you will always be human. No matter how much you let yourself be fucked, fisted, beaten, shat on, or whatever, or how much you do it yourself, your mind will always be there, telling your body whether or not it's turned on. Better accept it.

If you can manage that, then you can enjoy yourself in the depths of the beast and experience mind-blowing pleasure. Being aware that you are exchanging intimacies as a man with another man does, after all, have a mentally hot aspect, namely that he is in some way

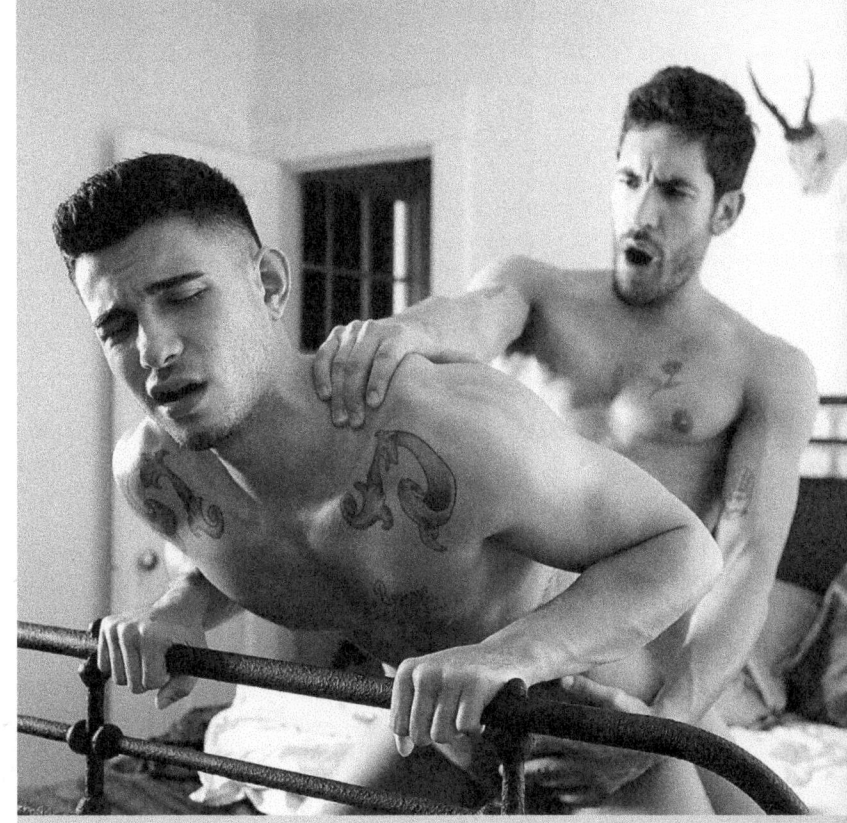

May there be peace and goodwill on earth.

revealing himself to you. He is showing you his desires, his lust, and sharing them with you.

In doing this, he is also revealing to you part of his mind, his soul, for instance, in the way he presents or receives sex. No matter how deeply you wallow with him in the pits of animal lust, looking into his eyes will always reveal his mind. The longing for union with this man will always be greater than its fulfillment, but experiencing it together can be satisfying enough, if it happens on the same level. That can happen while you're fucking, fisting, beating, or shitting on him. It can also happen in a kiss. If you know the feeling of never being full or never being hungry, please be aware of the wonderful gift you have been given: the gift of having sex with another man. It is a universal gift, even though the wrapping may vary. A meeting of man and man. Amen.

Although I'm not religious, I have found it helpful to see myself as part of a larger whole, in the sense of mankind, the earth, the universe, creation. I generally find everyone interesting, but I would rather spend time with those that are pleasantly interesting rather than those who try to be unpleasantly interesting.

If you are able to create your own mental sexual universe, then even a kiss, or an exchange of glances with another man can be a sexual climax. That doesn't mean you can't plunge into your filthiest depths with him. But you don't have to.

On the one hand, we seek reconciliation with our animal lusts—which may make us feel guilty and immoral—on the other we strive for the spiritual, the godly. The animal part of ourselves is part of the universe, it is one of its aspects.

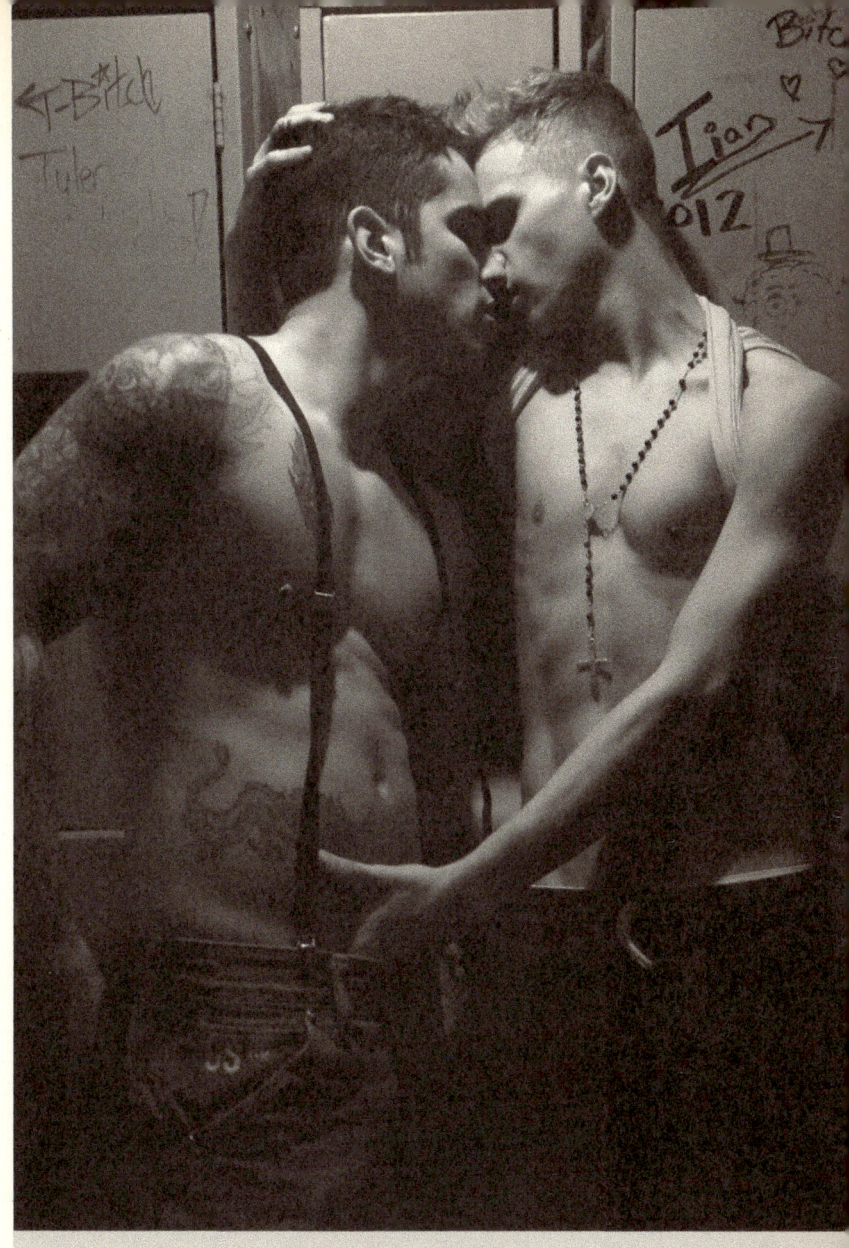

"Show me what you've got—and not just in your pants."

Four Steps to Nirvana?

As we mentioned in the beginning, the time needed to carry out a sexual act is not necessarily a criteria for its quality. With the right consciousness, focused on what is happening right now, even a quickie can give you quite a kick. But in any case, good sex means that one partner's body and mind are attuned to that of the other partner. For a quickie, the chatting and flirting leading up to the act itself may form the basis for an intense encounter. What's the next step?

▼ Do Me Quickly

Personally, I will never be able to understand the mental and emotional state necessary to be sexually aroused—to say nothing of climaxing through pain, humiliation, or submission—without a long warming-up period. There is no question that this exists, but probably only where there's a certain routine and an absolute awareness of each person's needs. Then you can get right down to business: three slaps on the ass and the sap will rise!

After all, everyone has experienced a brief encounter that made us happy. But how to turn a quickie into a memorably hot experience? You need either an unforgettably attractive guy—maybe a celebrity, as who would ever forget a hook-up with Keanu Reeves?—or an unforgettably adventurous setting. My top three quickies fall into this category, probably due to my continuing lack of celebrity action. (Call me, Mr. Reeves!)

▶ Third place: In the Night Train from Paris to Munich (Sleeping Car)

After a brief chat with a nice Frenchman, we both slipped into our bunks, which were at the bottom of the compartment, next to each other. Above us were two unoccupied bunks, then an elderly lady and a teenaged girl, who went straight to sleep. We, however, got closer to one another in the darkness until the Frenchman eventually crept into my bunk and there was a short but thrilling interlude. Early next morning, he woke me and got off the train. We exchanged addresses and he wrote me a letter expressing his delight in our successful little adventure. So I had proof, as in hindsight I could hardly believe it myself.

▶ Second place: In a Night Train from Kassel to Frankfurt (Second Class Compartment)

On the train home one night, famished after a week's service in the army, I spied a sexy young guy sitting alone in the compartment. Rather brashly, I tried to pick up the man who was reading a newspaper and was surprised myself when it actually worked! Without

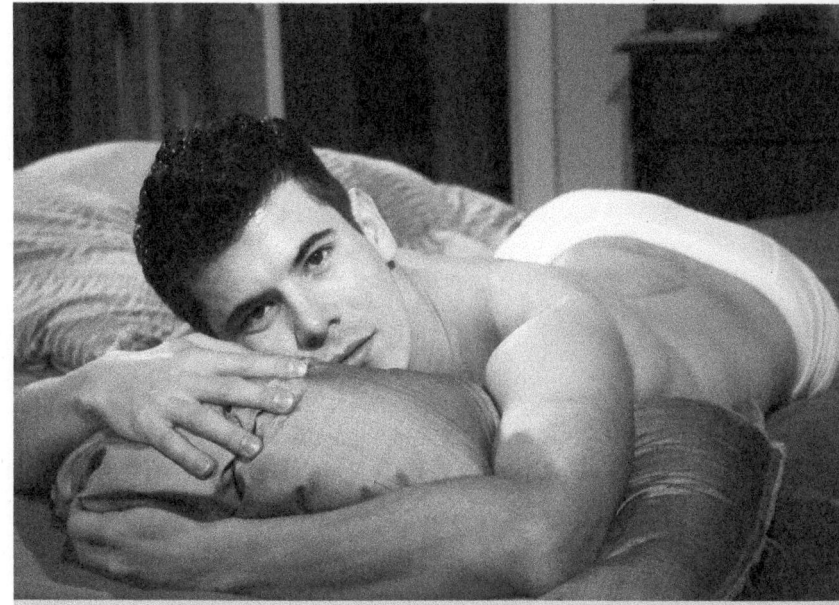

Alone in the sleeper car, ready for action

further ado, he closed the curtains, we stripped naked and enjoyed a nervous, but due to the attendant circumstances, exciting tryst. I still miss the compartments of those old InterCity trains!

▶ **First place: In the Crowd of Spectators During the July 14th—the French National Holiday-Parade (Paris)**

While my friends were attentively watching the parade, I could barely respond to their comments. The roaming hands of a cheeky French tyke standing right in front of me required the utmost concentration, for after a brief glance at me and a dizzying smile, he made a grab for my pants. *Oh, là, là!* So dexterous was he that no one noticed anything at all, and afterwards he tidily sorted my crown jewels back where they belonged. Once the crowd had dispersed after the parade was over, he stood waiting with his buddies and shot me a grin. I could barely tear myself away, and my friends laughed themselves sick when I told them why. *L'amour, l'amour, l'amour!*

▼ **Do Me Right**

Whether you're doing right by a guy, or whether he's doing you right, will make itself known to you in the middle. Not at the beginning, not at the end, but in between. It doesn't last long, but it doesn't need to, it's enough if the right feeling flares up a couple of times. Even if you employ all the physical sophistication in the world, the pathway always runs via the head, via the mind. This is always the goal. Glances, words, the way you touch each other, all of this leads to the really crucial erotic stimulation and creates its own movie. You yourself will sense it somewhere in your spinal cord or your brain, that hot bolt of lightning that will go on illuminating the memory of this experience for a long time.

Your partner can only give you this experience if you've allowed him to get close enough to you to have an idea of what you want. It's

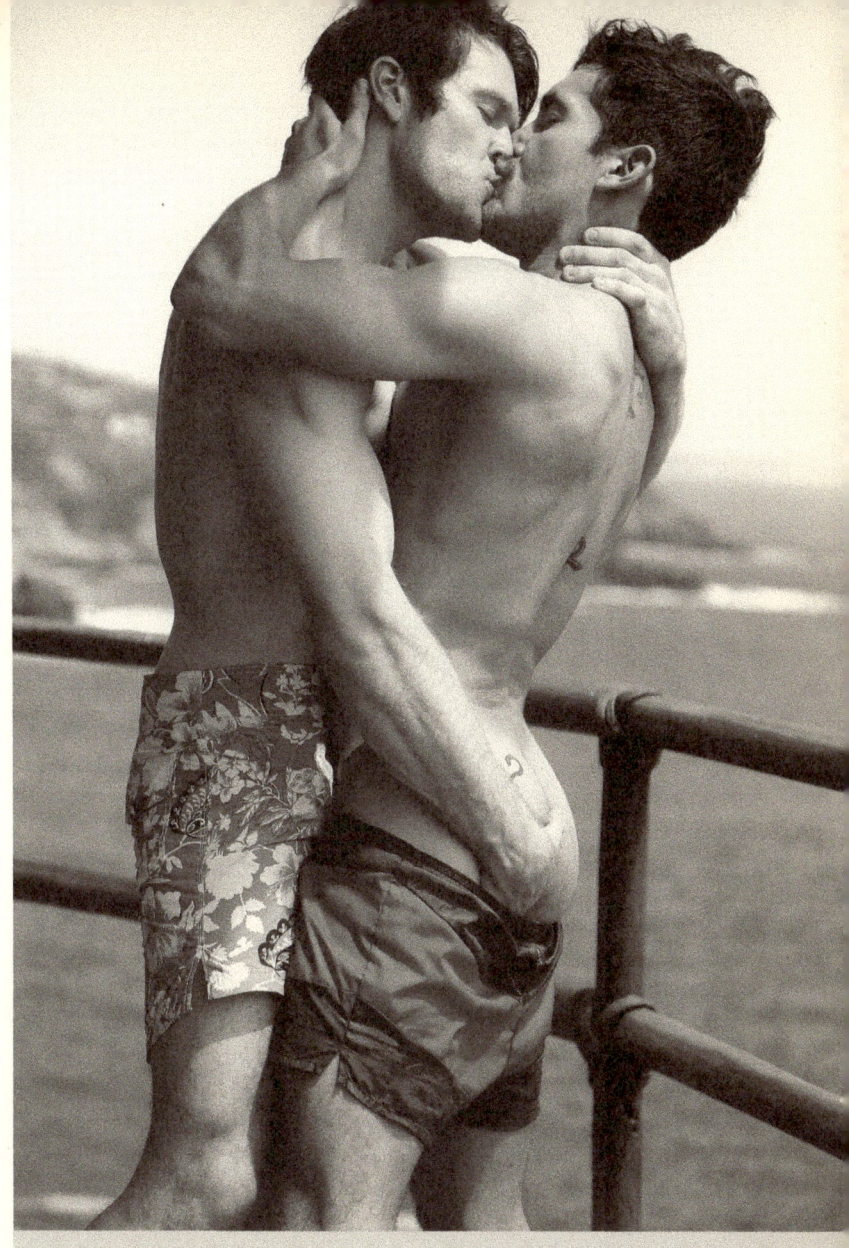

A little PDA never hurt anyone.

enough to show him that you're open to his fantasies, it's enough to make him feel welcome. You can garnish your filthy-brute act with a wink, your cute-but-bratty persona with an inviting smile.

Once the fire has been lit, a burst of sparks can rain down on both of you. Whoever feels it first will pass it on, like an Olympic flame.

You can ignite the flames by creating the right conditions for your own personal sexual high and then touching your partner with fire, carrying him along. How quickly you spur each other onwards depends on the amount of time you want it to take.

And then you can bring that really sexy combination into play: focusing on individual senses and stimuli, not confining yourself to one topic but rather involving the entire body. The opposition between standstill and motion, dominance and submission, egotism and empathy, pleasure and pain. And then let him see a tiny glimpse of your mind behind these sheer animal spirits—wow! If only I could have really good sex more often!

▼ Do Me Fancy

Unless you're a master of empathy, or have found one, you can't get terribly fancy and sophisticated until you've actually gotten to know your partner. As a rule, you shouldn't get too fancy on a first, or even on a second or third date, as your success will be determined by your knowledge of—or at least a feeling for—what methods to use. But you have to find that out beforehand. That's why having a steady partner or fuck buddy represents the best opportunity for doing more than just letting off steam. Looking forward to sex, getting in the mood for it, dating or flirting, the clearer you make your positions, the better it will work out. Surprises should increase your pleasure, not distract from it, so you need to be able to gauge your partner's reaction. It's not the same thing as routine.

Sophisticated sex transcends the bodily experience, it is a work of art that can take you on a trip into your deepest desires. Your body is an instrument with which you can tickle the mind using any means. Costumes, role-play, toys, fluids, smells, dirt, pain, whatever floats your boat, it's all there in your box of tricks. But the real trick is a magic spell you have to come up with yourself—a new one for every time.

▼ Do Me Completely (and Utterly)

You can't have sex all night and all day. Your appetite is usually larger than your stomach. If you just race from one man to the next, from one adventure to the next, you might as well see sex as nothing but a means for propagating your genetic material. The desire for nonstop sex, whether in the insertive or in the receptive role, is difficult to reconcile with real life because everybody will start to flag at some point. Even if you have a 24-7 relationship, it's not always focused on sex, as we saw in the interview with Herrmeistersir.

Sometimes it just isn't that easy to get closer to one's goal of being "well and truly fucked." Sex, done properly, is always tiring, generally in a good way. Having really good sex once in a while—and a couple of quickies in between times, as long as you relish it—should be perfectly sufficient. Apart from that, your whole life can be sexy if you are turned on by the men around you, if you like to look at them—and perhaps you might get a look back. Forget about doing anyone completely!

Concluding Thoughts

> *Ten kisses are more easily forgotten than one.*
> *—Jean Paul*

I have nothing against vanilla sex. I love vanilla, cuddles, and flowers. But if I remember correctly, flowers don't really have sex with each other unless there's a bee involved. And that sting is what's sometimes missing in our love life.

It took courage for me to write this book. Who would want to claim to be an authority on sex? But then I realized that that isn't necessary at all. But then what is? I enjoy sex because once in a while I meet someone whose frequency I can become attuned to and who will come with me on a journey. A short one, a long one, or even a really long one. I am curious, I like to experiment, but I do have boundaries. I am aware of a number of them. Whenever my imagination fails me, I look forward to being inspired by other men who have often fired my own imagination so that I make their fantasies my own.

That's the reason why I decided to write this book: It's actually just about the stories. The stories I tell here are meant to inspire you, no more and no less. Plenty of people could tell them, maybe better than me, plenty of people already have, after all there are all kinds of gay sex stories out there, but that's not the point either. Now I've done it myself too and offered my own suggestions that you, the reader, can fill with your own ideas and images.

While in my opinion, there are a lot of universal truths in this book, aside from all the half-truths, it is really up to you to decide what is true or false, and whether or not you agree with me.

Thank you for the trust you have placed in me by reading this book.

Many thanks also to Peter, Darryl, Olaf, Fred, Herrmeistersir, Hilmar, Tommy, Noé, Rainer, Andreas, and Roland.

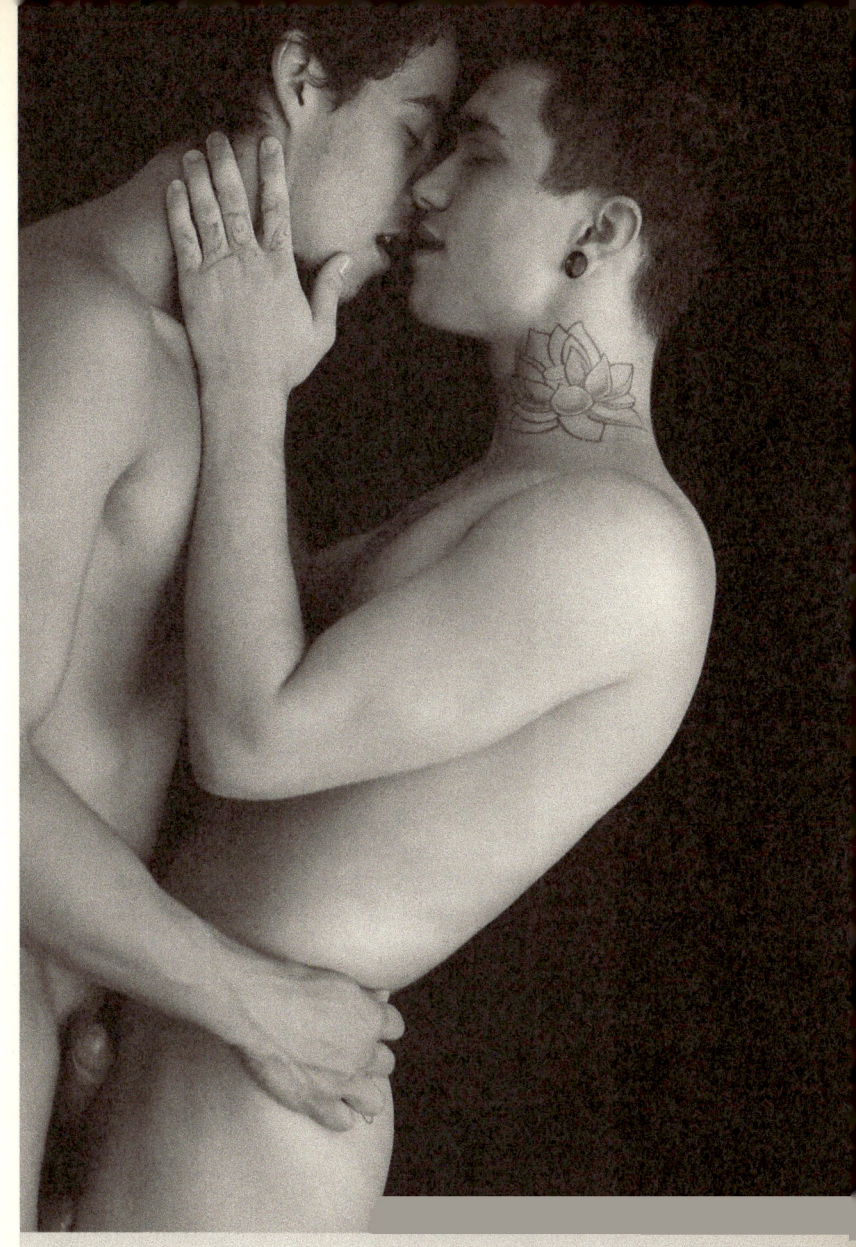

Intimacy comes in many forms.

Safer Sex

Safer sex with respect to HIV includes practices where there is no contact between blood or semen and mucous membranes or open wounds. Pay close attention to any cuts and abrasions on your skin, whether you're having normal intercourse or engaging in rough play. The rougher the play, the greater the wear and tear on your tissues will be, and so you need to reckon with injuries, even if you can't see them. If you injure your mouth, dick, or anus, this can lead to an exchange of blood or semen. If you are HIV positive, your blood and semen contain the highest concentration of viruses, so this can be enough infect your partner with HIV. Keeping this point in mind, the following practices with regard to HIV infections count as

▶ low risk/safe:

- ▶ stroking
- ▶ kissing
- ▶ slapping
- ▶ spitting
- ▶ pissing
- ▶ shitting
- ▶ fucking with a rubber (as long as your using a water-based lube—oil and other greasy lubricants such as Crisco can create tiny tears in the condom, making it unsafe)
- ▶ dildo play (always use a condom when switching from one partner to another)
- ▶ fisting with gloves

▶ presumably safe:

- ▶ blow jobs (as long as there is no semen in the urethra—for example, if it's been rinsed out shortly beforehand by peeing. Take it out before you cum! If you do come into contact with semen: spit, don't swallow!)

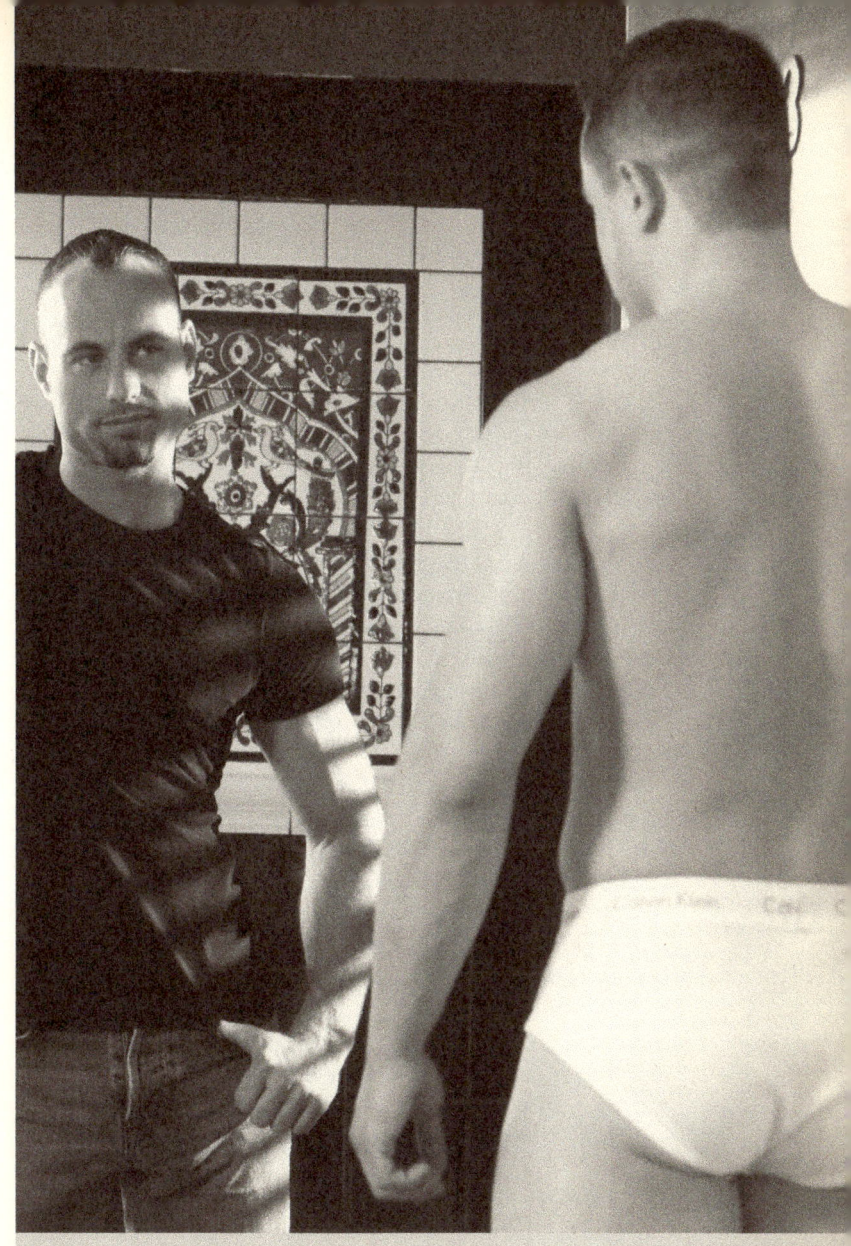

"Hi, neighbor. Have you come to do me?"

- swallowing saliva
- swallowing pre-cum
- rimming
- drinking piss
- eating shit

high risk/unsafe:

- taking semen in your mouth (the viruses in the fluid remain active following ejaculation)
- fucking without a rubber
- fisting without gloves

The viral load is especially high in HIV-positive people who aren't being treated at the moment or at all. You yourself could be highly contagious if you are unaware of your HIV status. AIDS can only be held in check if everyone is aware of his HIV infection and seeks treatment before the virus is passed on to other people through its high concentration in the blood or semen.

Contact with urine and feces carries the risk of a hepatitis infection. Vaccinations are available against hepatitis types A and B. As a rule, most doctors will recommend being inoculated against hepatitis, so asking for a vaccination will not give rise to any suspicions and requires no explanation. There is no vaccination for hepatitis type C. This disease is transmitted via the blood, so practices such as fisting without gloves are especially high-risk.

That leaves us with other sexually transmitted infections such as syphilis or gonorrhea. The bacteria can be transmitted via the saliva, pre-cum, urine, or feces. With a timely diagnosis, treatment is relatively uncomplicated and generally successful.

The best way of getting a handle on STIs is to have them treated as soon as possible, so that you don't spread them. So, if you notice any changes in your genitals or anywhere else on your body, go straight to a doctor you can trust before you embark on your next sexual adventure. Inform your latest sex partners of your diagnosis and give them the chance to have themselves examined and, if need be, treated.

On that note: Enjoy your amazing sexy life!

Photo credits:

▶ **Berlinmale.com:**
14, 68, 110, 115

▶ **Jake Jaxson & R J Sebastian (photographers) for CockyBoys.com:**
39, 55, 112, 134-135, 147, 153, 155, 159, 163

▶ **HotHouse.com:**
13, 16, 21, 34, 36, 42, 48, 51, 53, 58, 63, 66, 71, 80, 83, 98, 121, 123, 139, 144, 165, 157

▶ **LucasEntertainment.com:**
24, 32, 79, 89, 91, 94

▶ **Spritzz.com:**
19, 27, 75, 86, 109, 116

Everything a Man Needs to Know

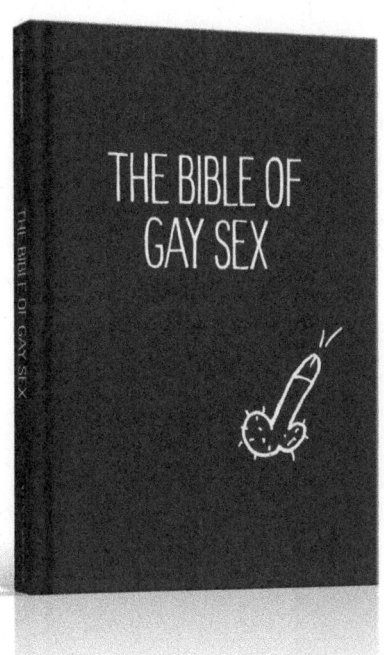

Guidebooks for the Curious and Adventurous

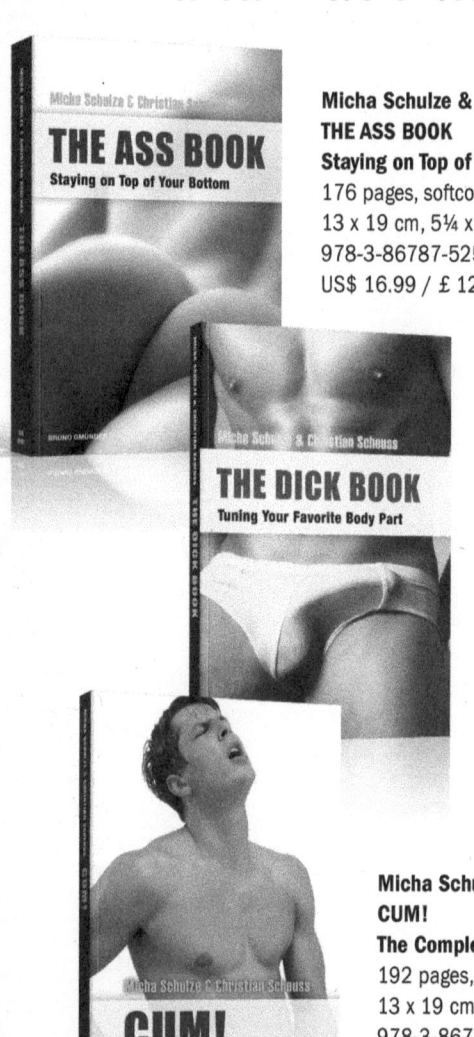

Micha Schulze & Christian Scheuss
THE ASS BOOK
Staying on Top of Your Bottom
176 pages, softcover,
13 x 19 cm, 5¼ x 7½",
978-3-86787-525-7
US$ 16.99 / £ 12.99 / € 14,95

Micha Schulze &
Christian Scheuss
THE DICK BOOK
Tuning Your Favorite Body Part
184 pages, softcover,
13 x 19 cm, 5¼ x 7½"
978-3-86787-446-5
US$ 15.99 / £ 11.99 / € 14,95

Micha Schulze & Christian Scheuss
CUM!
The Complete Guide to Orgasm
192 pages, softcover
13 x 19 cm, 5¼ x 7½"
978-3-86787-588-2
US$ 16.99 / £ 12,99 / € 14,95

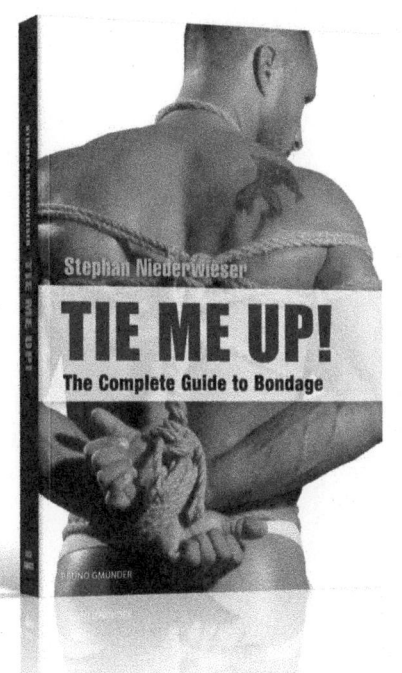

Stephan Niederwieser
TIE ME UP!
The Complete Guide to Bondage
256 pages, softcover,
17 x 24 cm, 5¼ x 7½"
ISBN 978-3-86787-599-8
US$ 32.99 / € 24,95

Bondage for everybody: Stephan Niederwieser's relaxed style and focus on pleasure are the perfect combination for this introduction to bondage, a book that's sure to benefit both the rank beginner and the experienced practitioner. Here you'll find everything you need to know about the most important toys and accessories, about different kinds of knots and how to tie them securely. You'll find all the tools you need to let go of your inhibitions and get the biggest bang from your bondage experience.

Gay Erotica at Its Best

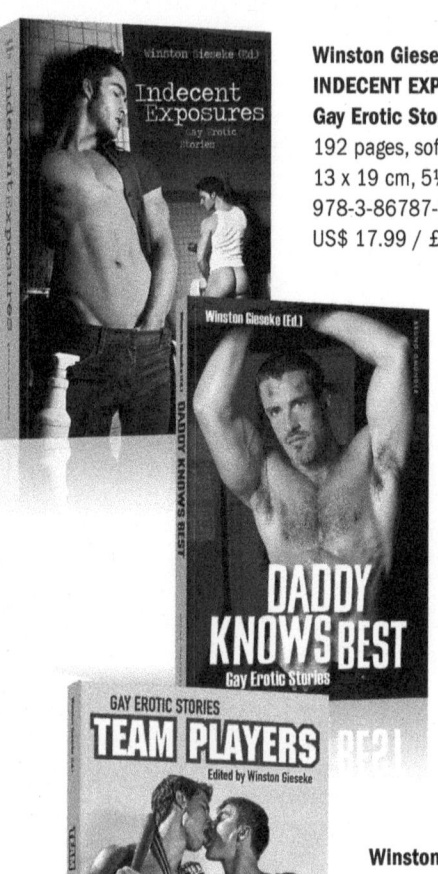

Winston Gieseke (Ed.)
INDECENT EXPOSURES
Gay Erotic Stories
192 pages, softcover,
13 x 19 cm, 5¼ x 7½",
978-3-86787-520-2
US$ 17.99 / £ 11.99 / € 16,95

Winston Gieseke (Ed.)
DADDY KNOWS BEST
Gay Erotic Stories
208 pages, softcover
13 x 19 cm, 5¼ x 7½"
978-3-86787-590-5
US$ 17.99 / £ 11.99 / € 15,95

Winston Gieseke (Ed.)
TEAM PLAYERS
Gay Erotic Stories
208 pages, softcover
13 x 19 cm, 5¼ x 7½"
978-3-86787-609-4
US$ 17.99 / £ 11.99 / € 15,95

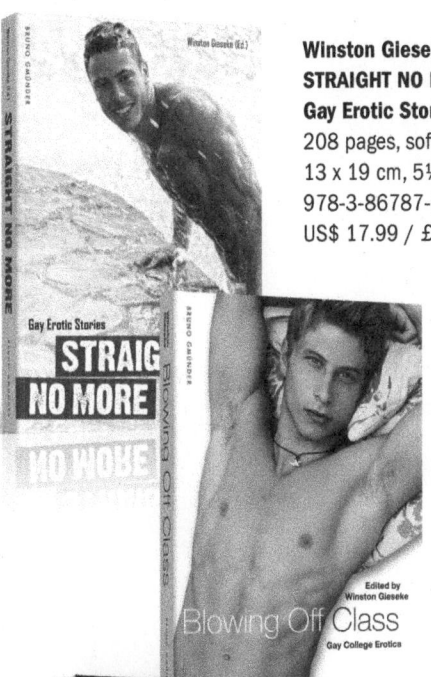

Winston Gieseke (Ed.)
STRAIGHT NO MORE
Gay Erotic Stories
208 pages, softcover,
13 x 19 cm, 5¼ x 7½",
978-3-86787-607-0
US$ 17.99 / £ 11.99 / € 16,95

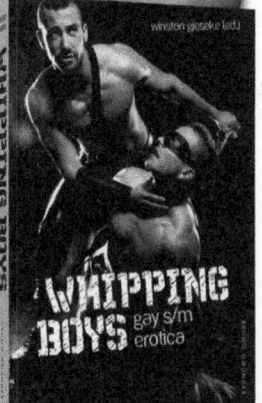

Winston Gieseke (Ed.)
BLOWING OFF CLASS
Gay Erotic Stories
208 pages, softcover
13 x 19 cm, 5¼ x 7½"
978-3-86787-686-5
US$ 17.99 / £ 11.99 / € 15,95

Winston Gieseke (Ed.)
WHIPPING BOYS
Gay S/M Erotica
208 pages, softcover
13 x 19 cm, 5¼ x 7½"
978-3-86787-689-6
US$ 17.99 / £ 11.99 / € 15,95

Release April 2014

Model: Jake Bass

COCKYBOYS.COM

Angel Rock

#fallenangel

HOT HOUSE
.com

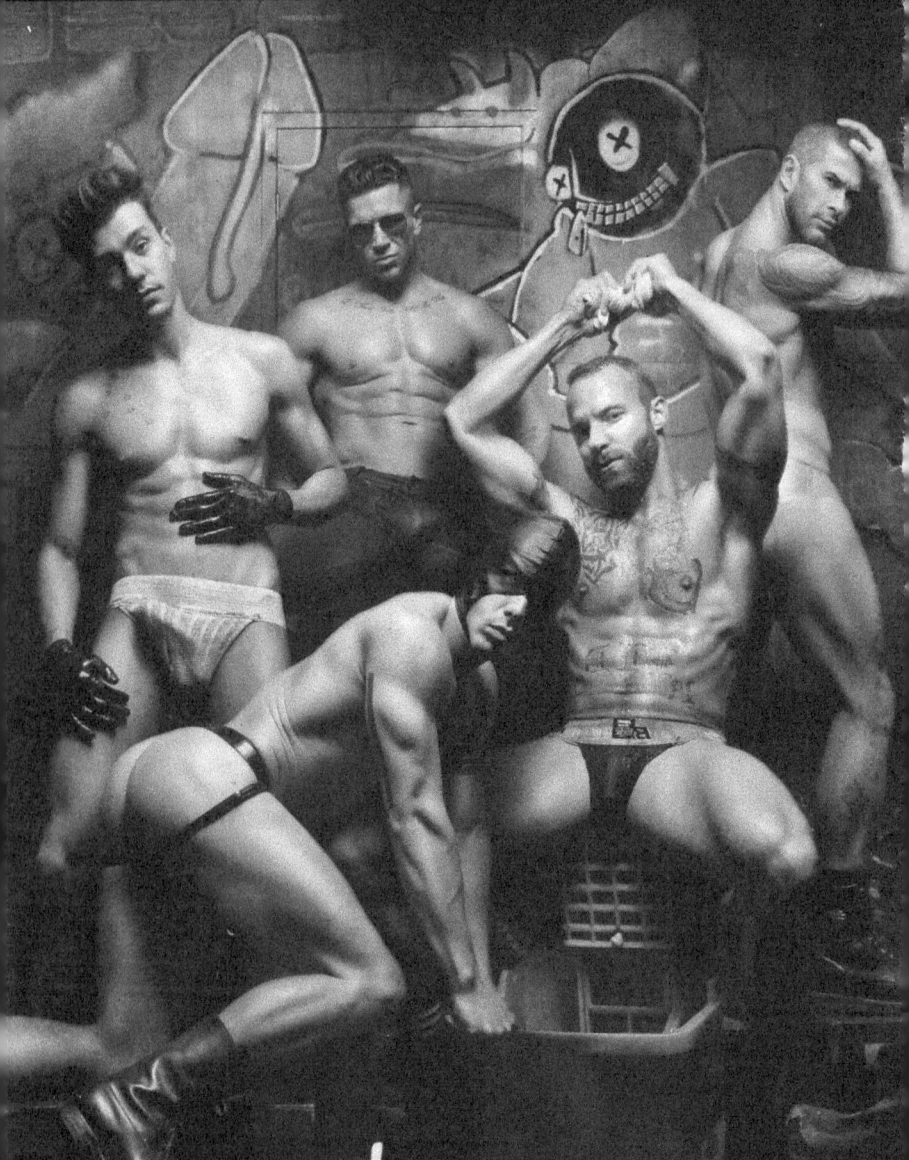

HARDER. FASTER. ROUGHER